I would like to dedicate this book to my son, Joseph Garland, for his continued support and belief in my ability to write; and to my aunt, Lucille, who always wanted to write, but didn't.

Jordan
Living with Autism and Multiple Complex Developmental Disorder
A Guide for the Rest of Us

Brenda Clemons

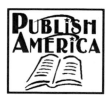

PublishAmerica
Baltimore

First printing

ISBN: 1-4241-8328-6
PUBLISHED BY PUBLISHAMERICA, LLLP
www.publishamerica.com
Baltimore

Printed in the United States of America

Acknowledgments

I would like to thank Dr. Yasser Ad-dab'bing, assistant professor of psychiatry at the University of Ottawa, for his kind giving of his time and knowledge in attempting to shed light on the mysteries of multiple complex developmental disorder.

Contents

Me

My life is so beautiful
by the world around me.
It is so nice living by
the deep blue sea.
It is so wonderful
and magical.
With dragons and
good dragons and
bad dragons.
And this world is so wonderful that
I have to live inside a beautiful home with
dogs, cats, sheep, and goats.
And I am a princess but
nobody knows.
And I am so gentle that is why
when I grow up I am going to go out and
find a prince and marry him.
Even then I am going to
walk the forest.
Even then I am going to
have army knights.
Even I am going to capture
dragons and
save them.
Oh! Man!

Written by Jordan, an eight-year-old girl diagnosed with autism and multiple complex developmental disorder.

Foreword

Autism is a mysterious condition that still mystifies scientists, doctors, and researchers. The parent of the autistic child is burdened with enough grief just dealing with their child: the unusual behaviors, the silence, the temper outbursts, the dreams that may never be fulfilled, and the desperation to hear their child say just one little word or sound—something, anything, that can keep alive the parent's hope that their child may someday "wake up," "snap out of it" or otherwise be healed. The grief that parents feel is compounded by the guilt a parent naturally feels when something is wrong with their child. It must be inherent in our biology, or even our souls, to need to protect and nurture our offspring. When something goes wrong and the child is born with an abnormality or spirals backwards into autism, it is only natural for the parent to feel that they are somehow responsible—that they have failed in the greatest task known to mankind—re-creation. We feel that if we fail our own offspring then we also fail ourselves. There is no greater pain than that of a parent who must sit and watch their child suffer. Our instincts to protect are enraged and our minds search for answers about the injustice and suffering that has been laid upon us and our children.

Even worse is the emotional suffering of the parent whose child has a mental illness. Society turns its face against the ugliness in itself. History is filled with accounts of cruelty put upon those suffering from mental illness: ancient civilizations believed that the mentally ill were possessed by demons and would attempt to "cure" the victim by cutting a whole in the victim's skull; and in recent modern times the mentally ill were made to endure lobotomies and electric shock therapy—all in the name of science and medicine. In the past psychoanalysts put much of the blame on childhood trauma. Autism was once thought to be caused by so-called "refrigerator mothers" who withheld affection from their children. It has been my experience that, even though found to be a flawed theory, the concept of bad parenting causing mental illness is still in the minds of many.

Now, imagine the struggles of a single mother whose child has been diagnosed with both autism and a form of psychosis; and not just any psychosis, but one that most people in North America have never heard of. Not only has it never been heard of, but there is much controversy over whether the child even has autism at all because research suggests that the condition only exhibits autism-like symptoms. How does the parent teach others about their child's condition if there is little known about it? Just receiving a proper diagnosis can take years due to the fact that most doctors are not properly trained on how to recognize and treat it.

The school system is inevitably unqualified to meet the needs of such children. Anything that challenges the system to "think out of the box" is met with not only resistance but distrust and suspicion. The fault does not lie solely with the teachers and school administrators; but with federal regulations. The "No Child Left Behind" act has left behind the children who need it the most—those with the greatest learning disabilities. Public schools are so busy worrying about federal regulations that they have begun to see children, not as individuals, but as numbers: test scores, IQ's, and government grants that can be withheld if the school does not meet government standards of learning.

When I first set out to write this book my sole purpose was to write a book full of commonsense advice and information. In the process something amazing happened. Jordan started to speak her mind. She said the words and I attempted to type fast enough to keep up with her train of thought. In doing this I found real gems. I now know that Jordan is full of deep thoughts and is probably, in many ways, more mature than most children her age. My idea of a simple book grew into something bigger—to give a voice to Jordan so that others may see the beauty that she holds inside; so that others may see her as not just a number, but as an individual with unique ideas.

I wish that I could close this book in a nice tidy manner—with a happy ending. Unfortunately, in the reality of autism and mental illness there is no such thing. The best that we, the parents of such children, can hope for is the strength to continue on in our struggle for justice, scientific research, understanding, and education. If we are lucky, each day we see a glimpse of the divine in our children—which gives us the hope we need in order to carry on.

Introduction

My name is Jordan. I am artistic. I love horses. I go to a special class that is for artistic children. And I ride horses. Horses is my favorite animal. I have three dogs actually, who is one dog is Mac, the other dog is Henry, the other dog is Taco. I like to do write in my writing tablet when I have a chance to. My favorite thing in the whole wide world. I love my mommy who is strong person and who is writing this book about me, Jordan Clemons. And I love her. I always wanted a horse, a flying unicorn horse, all my life. But it won't come true cause I have to wait for what my mom is doing. I love mommy. I am artistic and my mommy is writing how to take care of artistic children. She always gets most of the time but I love her but her always forgives me and I love her.

—Jordan

Jordan is an eight-year-old girl. She is a first-grade student who loves math, playing with other children, and drawing. She struggles with phonics even though she loves books. Her favorite TV show is the *Power Rangers* (when she is allowed to watch it). She loves horses and goes horseback riding about once a week. She takes ballet but hates wearing her tights. Her obsession at the moment is advancing in her Super Mario video game (which she plays on her Nintendo DS). On the surface, it would seem that, relatively speaking, Jordan is just like every other child in the United States, but she is not; Jordan has been diagnosed with autism and underlying multiple complex developmental disorder.

Because of her disorder, Jordan cannot speak clearly. While I can understand about 70 to 80 percent of her speech, people outside of our family say they can only understand about 45 to 50 percent of what she is saying. Jordan loves to play with other children but is afraid to approach them and will ask me to approach children for her. Jordan becomes frustrated easily because she does not know how to interact with her peers. She goes to ballet once a week, but she does not interact with her classmates, and it appears that they have learned not to interact with her. She is a wiz at math and already knows how to add and subtract, but she still does not know her alphabet or how to read.

While most children have temper tantrums, Jordan's tantrums become violently out of control. During the past 18 months she has strangled me, broken my nose, and bitten her social worker. The reason for her behavior is now apparent, however, at the age of six we did not know she is autistic. As Jordan's mother, of course I knew something was wrong, but I am not a doctor and I had no choice but to go on the advice I was being given by the "experts" who told me that my daughter was simply developmentally delayed. When I raised my concern about her speech, I was told that she merely had a speech impairment and that a bit of speech therapy was all she needed to improve.

It became increasingly hard to get Jordan to go to school. She even jumped out of a moving car in order to avoid school. As a result of her refusal, a host of social workers and other mental health workers became involved. I was told that Jordan had separation anxiety and that I could not control my daughter. The advice they gave me resulted in Jordan's behavior spiraling out of control. Finally, at the end of my breaking point, I quite my job and homeschooled her.

The Board of Education filed charges against me for truancy and child abuse and neglect. It took five court hearings, three lawyers, three social workers, and $1,500 to get the matter cleared up.

In spite of all the hardships, I do not regret any of it. Jordan is a joy to have around. She is intelligent, caring, and creative. I have grown tremendously as a result of having her in my life. I am also a much wiser person.

My wish is to not just share Jordan's story, but to also educate the public, to share the wisdom that I have acquired, and to bring hope and knowledge to other parents who are now finding themselves in similar situations.

Brenda Clemons

Chapter 1

Characteristics of Children with Autism and MCDD

Hello, my name is Jordan Clemons. I am artistic. I am seven years old. My mommy is trying to figure out what it is like to be artistic, well, here it is. There is defferent of, of, like, of, like artistic. There is where, is one where you can't talk. And there is another one, what I have is where I can talk. But I am mad and throw stuff and everything, And there is another one where you can talk but you don't feel comfortable with everything. And most of time you know what he is talking about. And there is another one where you is nice.

Here is what it is like, I don't like lights and I go crazy. The lights hurt my eyes so bad that I go crazy and I yell at people. And I don't like loud screeching noises. It feels like I just want to take my fist and punch it into a wall. And that is how I feel like. Sometimes I like to be alone. 'Cause sometime I get mad and I like to be alone outside riding my bike. And I always like to do the monkey bars at school. But sometimes it is difficult for me because when I come in, I have to say hello to my teachers and hang up

*my coat and book bag and even I read and even then I do some
activities but I also need to check my schedule I am scared to
approach them 'cause of I am afraid to talk to them and to speak
to them and I don't know if they understand me. I need help and
sometimes when I can read and I look at the words and then I can
find the same words but I am very good at that because of my
teacher is there to help me with it and I am autistic.*

—Jordan (on what it's like to be autistic)

Jordan loved her pre-kindergarten class. Her day was filled with
music and exercises designed for the slow learner. Her teacher was
very kind and Jordan talked affectionately about her.

In kindergarten Jordan was put into a regular classroom with 35 other
children. The classroom had one teacher and one assistant. Jordan went
to a special education teacher for reading and math. It was at this point
that Jordan's bizarre behaviors became increasingly evident. The stress
of the large classroom full of noisy children was just too much for her.

Her teachers did not have the time that is required to teach and care
for a child like Jordan. Their inability became apparent when Jordan
took a baby tooth to school for "show and tell." The tooth was
misplaced and it took almost six weeks to find it.

Jordan knew exactly where her tooth was all along (in her cubby
hole). The problem seems to be that her teachers failed to understand
her and did not take the time to try and understand. Her lost tooth
became a big issue for Jordan. I finally solved her problem by going
into her classroom before the start of the school day to search for her
tooth. It was right where she said it would be.

Characteristics of Autism and MCDD

While the symptoms of autism and multiple complex
developmental disorder can vary greatly from child to child, there are
some common characteristics that are apparent and easily spotted.

Characteristics of Autism

• Inability to withstand normal environmental stimuli.
• Inability to communicate normally. May not be able to speak at all.
• Will make stuttering noises or other unusual and/or repetitive sounds.
• Must have a strict routine. Inability to handle changes in daily schedule
• Appears to be off in their own world
• Inability to cope with close human contact (such as hugging).
• Attachment to unusual objects (such as kitchen gadgets).
• Inability to or resistance to playing with other children
• Lack of imagination
• Sudden and explosive bursts of anger.
• Repetitive behaviors
• Unusual fascination with things that spin (such as wheels)
• May have some skill that seems to be above current IQ level.
• Fascination with putting objects in a straight line.

Characteristics of Children with MCDD

• Intense anxiety
• Social detachment
• Thought processes well out of proportion with mental age
• Unusual fears
• Inability to initiate peer relationships
• Confusion between reality and fantasy
• Recurrent episodes of panic or terror
• Extreme attachments to parents, caregiver, or therapist. Positive behaviors may suddenly turn to episodes of aggressive or violent behavior towards these same people.
• Easily confused
• Delusions including an overactive fascination with fantasy figures.

• Inability to understand another person's pain or emotions.

• May have periods of uncontrolled laughter or giggling for no apparent reason.

Chapter 2

My name is Jordan. I am seven years old. I love horses all my life. I love to go to school. We always have snack time before lunch. But today I am having popcorn and Gatorade. Even I like my school bus. I always ride it when I got to school but the days my mom picks me up for an appointment. So I am packing up my video games so I can have something to do. And my mom tells my school she is picking me up today. Even I always write on my writing tablet because I love to. And I am a smart cookie (laughter). But I am in music class. I go to art class and speech cause of that is the only class I go to right now. Even I am going to my class after everything so I can write on my school writing tablet for a little while. And that is it.

—Jordan (on her school day)

I moved my family to a county which has much more resources for children with disabilities. At the time I hoped that this move would result in Jordan improving her attitude about school. I was frustrated when her behaviors not only continued, but escalated out of control. She started jumping out of my moving automobile as I attempted to drive her to school. It was at this point that Jordan said that an adult, a non-family member, had touched her inappropriately.

I reported this to the authorities. It is unfortunate that her allegations were declared unfounded. I cannot help but think that the outcome would have been a bit different if Jordan did not have the disability that she does.

A Brief History

The word autism was coined from the Greek word autos— meaning self. Dr. Leo Kanner, a child psychologist at John Hopkins University, first used the word in the 1940s. At the time he was working with a group of children whose abilities varied widely. Some of these children could talk but most could not. Those who did talk usually were not able to effectively communicate their thoughts. The children could not show affection, and most would have episodes of extreme violence. This group of children also demonstrated repetitive behaviors such as hand flapping and rocking back and forth. Dr. Kanner's work was groundbreaking and, thus, opened up the study of autism.

Also doing research around the same time as Dr. Kanner was the Australian psychologist Dr. Hans Asperger. Dr. Asperger was busy working with a group of children who had symptoms similar to those of the children being studied by Dr. Kanner, except the children Dr. Asperger was studying had several marked differences: these children had relatively high IQ's, they could communicate well and usually had verbal skills beyond those of their peers. The term Asperger syndrome was not used to describe high-functioning autistic children until 1981.

In the late 1940s, Dr. Bruno Bettelheim published his refrigerator mom theory. In his paper, Dr. Bettelheim wrote that mothers who withheld physical affection and emotional support caused a type of psychosis to develop in their children. It is unfortunate that Dr. Bettelheim based his theory on watching children and adults in Nazi prison camps. His theories soon caught on and he became the most trusted autism authority of his time. The result being that autistic children were placed in mental institutions with no hope of improving.

Luckily, Richard Pollack did some research on Dr. Bettelheim. Pollack had a younger brother who was a patient at a facility run by Dr. Bettelheim and thus had a personal interest in Dr. Bettelheim and his work. Pollack found out that Dr. Bettelheim was not a doctor at all. Bettelheim, before immigrating to America, had worked in his family-owned lumber yard. His only college study was in art history. In short, Bettelheim had no qualifications to be a doctor or run a hospital. Thankfully, the era of seeing autism as a mental illness had come to an end.

In 1969, Anna Freud was working with children who were incapable of being soothed, had great anger outbursts, and poor reality testing. She coined these children "borderline." Fourteen years later, Simon Baron Cohen presented his theory that borderline children also showed symptoms of autism. Cohen's theory resulted in borderline children being lumped in with autistic children labeled under persuasive developmental disorder not otherwise specified (PDD, NOS). Researchers in the 1990s modified the criteria set forth by Cohen in order to come up with new criteria which they labeled "multiple complex developmental disorder." This term has been met with dispute in North America because researchers have found fault with the previous collection of data. Other countries, such as France and Switzerland, have readily accepted the term and are doing research on children who meet the MCDD criteria. Most of what is now known about behaviors and treatments has come from Dutch researchers. The fact that MCDD is not recognized in the United States is unfortunate but not a dead end. It is inevitable that it will soon be as common here as it is elsewhere in the world. Asperger's, which is now widely known and diagnosed in North America, was not included in the American Psychiatric Association's *Diagnostic and Statistical Manual of Mental Disorders* as a separate disorder until the fourth edition in 1994.

The study and treatment of autism came into the 21st century thanks to Dr. Bernard Rimland, Ph.D. Dr. Rimland has a son with autism, so the study of it is personal for him. Dr. Rimland has researched and published several studies that changed the world's understanding of autism, its causes, and its treatment. Dr. Rimland is the founder of the Autism Society of America (ASA). The ASA is the first organization developed to provide information and support to doctors and parents.

What Is Autism

Autism is defined as a condition which affects the brain, resulting in interference with communication, relationship, and social abilities. The result is that autistic children are overwhelmed by the world around them. While most of us might be vaguely aware of the noises coming form outside our window, an autistic child will hear them as clearly as they hear the television program they are watching.

Imagine, if you can, what it must be like when the smallest touch, the feel of the floor beneath your feet, the lights, everything in the environment around you, is all recognized by your brain as having equal importance. You would not be able to shut out anything. The normal brain categorizes our environment by importance. You, reading this book right now, are able to concentrate on the words on this page because your brain has prioritized these words as the most important thing. While you are reading this, there are probably various amounts of sound coming from the room next to yours. You may be aware of these sounds, but you are able to shut them out because your brain recognizes the sounds as being low on the importance scale. An autistic child does not have this ability.

Their senses are much more keen than those of a non-autistic person. Autistic children usually shy away from mud, paint, and other textures that they find distasteful; for example, Jordan will actually vomit if she comes in contact with play dough or finger paint.

In an effort to create some type of order and/or control, the autistic child will do things that the rest of us find strange, such as lining up objects, flapping their hands, or rocking back and forth.

Autistic children find it hard to communicate. Jordan can talk and communicate fairly well, but many children in her class do not. The inability to communicate added with the overwhelming amount of environmental stimuli (lighting, sounds, etc.) often results in meltdowns. Meltdowns are uncontrollable temper tantrums. It is believed that meltdowns are caused when things become just too much for the child to handle.

There is no typical autistic child. In fact, many researchers state that autism is as unique as a fingerprint, no two are exactly alike. Take, for example, the children in Jordan's class. Jordan can talk but will vomit if she comes in contact with paint, glue, or play dough. Richard can't talk at all, but he is the fastest in his class when it comes to putting together puzzles. Rachael obsessively lines up everything within her reach. She is mainstreamed in with non-autistic children for reading and math because of her high ability in these areas.

Many times parents mistake their children's hypersensitivity to certain stimuli as just misbehavior. Be aware when shopping with your artistic child. If they melt down every time you go out in public, it is probably the autism and not something your child can control. Try removing the child from the environment and see if that calms them down. Parents of autistic children must act carefully when correcting their child.

What Is Asperger's

Asperger's syndrome has most of the same symptoms as autism except for one major difference; Asperger's children usually have great communication skills. It is believed by many in the autism field that there are more Asperger's children than we know of. The reason being is that their symptoms are so mild, that parents and teachers assume that the child is just shy.

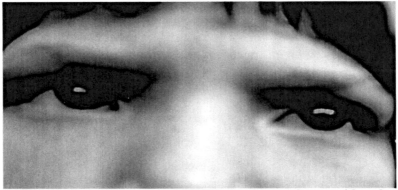

Research suggests that MCDD should not be considered a form of autism, but is its own unique condition.

What Is MCDD

Recently, there has been much debate in the medical field in regards to borderline syndrome, also known as multiple complex developmental disorder (MCDD). Practically unheard of, children with MCDD are typically just called PDD NOS. Or, they are not diagnosed as autistic at all, and are instead diagnosed with bipolar or another psychosis. The reason for the mental health diagnosis is because of the fascination with fantasy, and tendency towards violence that MCDD children typically have. Research suggests that 17 percent of children with MCDD manifest schizophrenia as adults, while 56 percent develop a schizophoid personality disorder.

Recent studies are suggesting that MCDD should not be lumped in with autism at all. Researchers are now suggesting that MCDD really is a unique condition, and as such, should be treated as one.

Jordan is easily confused between fantasy and reality. I am still learning how to differentiate between her pretend play and those times when her fantasies become her reality. Jordan loves dragons and our house is filled with dragon books. She recently found a rather large, smooth rock. She has decided that this is a dragon egg and has taken to sleeping with it. Luckily her books say that a dragon egg can take up to a 1,000 years to hatch; otherwise, I would be stuck trying to explain why her "egg" has not yet cracked open. In a humorous outcome to this story, I recently hired someone to do some yard work. This person somehow accidentally cut the rock in two. Jordan was extremely upset when she found her "egg" broken. In an effort to soothe her I suggested that perhaps the dragon had hatched and flown away. Jordan replied to me, "Mom! It was a rock; not a real dragon's egg. What, are you crazy?" With children like Jordan, you can never be sure what they are thinking—they will often surprise you.

Jordan has intense periods of anxiety and fear. Her most recent bout of fear centered around the thought that I would die if she ever left my side. Needless to say, it was a stressful period and she missed many days of school during this time. I am unsure just how long she has had this fear because the autism often interferes with her ability to tell me things. Usually, something has been going on for some time before Jordan is able to find a way to talk about it.

My challenge as a parent is learning what I can change about Jordan and what I need to just accept. At eight years old, Jordan sleeping with a dragon egg is rather cute. Jordan sleeping with a rock at the age of sixteen would be a problem. At what point do I try to explain to her that dragons don't really exist? Will she ever be able to accept it?

Dealing with Jordan and her disability has given me strength in character. One area of growth for me has been learning to love a child that is capable of causing me so much harm (broken noses, etc). It is a daily challenge to keep in mind that Jordan's aggression is a symptom of her disorder and not because she really does wish to hurt me.

Why Are They Grouped Together

During the recent past many names have been used to describe children with various degrees of autistic symptoms: autistic, Asperger's syndrome, high functioning, low functioning, multiple complex developmental disorder (MCDD), persuasive developmental disorder (PDD), and not other specified (NOS). If this sounds confusing, it's because it is. In an effort to make it easier for everyone, doctors started to lump all of autism into PDD or PDD NOS.

The drawback is that most autistic children do not conveniently fit into this category. The category is so wide that many children get lost in it and do not necessarily get all of the services they would otherwise qualify for. Often, doctors lump children (who may or may not be autistic) into the PDD NOS category simply because they don't know what else to call them.

If you are a parent with a child that has been lumped (or dumped) into the PDD NOS category, I strongly encourage you to keep at your child's doctors until you get a more precise diagnosis. A more precise diagnosis will give you more leverage when fighting for your child's legal rights in the educational system. It will also help with insurance purposes and getting your child the necessary referrals for various therapies and other treatments.

Interview with Dr. Yasser Ad-Dab'Bagh

Dr. Yasser Ad-Dab'Bagh is assistant professor of psychiatry at the University of Ottawa. He has written articles published in the *Journal of the American Academy of Child & Adolescent Psychiatry*, the *Canadian Journal of Psychiatry,* and is a contributor to the book *Does God Help? Developmental and Clinical Aspects of Religious Belief.* Please visit his website at www.publications.doctoraddabbagh.com and www.doctoraddabbagh.com

1. Introduce yourself and tell us a little about your background.

My name is Yasser Ad-Dab'bagh. I'm a child and adolescent psychiatrist, a psychoanalyst, and a researcher in the field of developmental neuroscience.

Currently, I'm an assistant professor of psychiatry at the University of Ottawa, and the psychiatrist on the Dual Diagnosis Team at the Children's Hospital of Eastern Ontario. The Dual Diagnosis Team specializes in the treatment of children and adolescents with highly complex clinical presentations that complicate either intellectual disability (ID) or pervasive developmental disorders (PDD, also referred to as autistic spectrum disorders, ASD).

I did my psychiatric and neuroscientific training at McGill University, where I continue to do research, and my psychoanalytic training at the Canadian Institute of Psychoanalysis. I'm a fellow of the Royal College of Physicians and Surgeons of Canada, a member of the Canadian Psychoanalytic Society and the International Psychoanalytical Association, a member of the Organization for Human Brain Mapping, a member of the Canadian Psychiatric Association and the American Psychiatric Association, and a member of the Canadian Academy of Child and Adolescent Psychiatry and the American Academy of Child and Adolescent Psychiatry.

My research interests are the normal and abnormal development of the human brain, brain-imaging, the regulation of the opioid receptors and endorphin system, developmental psychopharmacology, and the efficacy of attachment-based psychotherapeutic intervention.

2. For those who don't know, what is Multiple Complex Developmental Disorder? Is it a form of psychosis, a learning disability, or a form of autism?

Multiple-Complex Developmental Disorder (MCDD) is a term used by some child and adolescent psychiatrists to describe children and youth who have a particular set of complex symptoms. These symptoms are otherwise usually conceptualized as belonging to a number of coexisting conditions. However, due to what appears to be a consistent clustering of these symptoms, efforts were made to conceptualize them as belonging to a single syndrome.

This syndrome was initially called "the borderline syndrome of childhood." This term was influenced by the perception that these children were on the "border" of psychosis, but not quite psychotic. It was also influenced by the perception that these children's psychological development was likely to lead to substantial impairment in many domains of their life, in a manner similar to severe personality disorders.

When the apparent similarity to PDD of some of the symptoms of MCDD was noticed, a move towards conceptualizing it as a variant of PDD (ASD) led to the introduction of the term "Multiplex Developmental Disorder." This was later modified to Multiple-Complex Developmental Disorder. The experience clinicians have had with the patients that have met proposed criteria for MCDD, and the available literature describing neuropsychological and neurophysiological investigations of children with MCDD, support this diagnostic construct and suggest a degree of specificity.

In my opinion, the nosological construct of this disorder does not lend itself well to being included in either the PDDs or the personality disorders, and doesn't necessarily merit inclusion among the psychotic disorders. In other words, I do not conceptualize it as a form of autism, personality disorder, or psychosis. Instead, I feel it deserves to be in a category of its own. However, consensus about the validity of the construct, let alone the category of disorders it belongs to has not been reached in the psychiatric community. Although individuals with MCDD may have learning and/or other cognitive disabilities, MCDD itself is not a form of learning disability.

3. What are the symptoms of MCDD?

Unfortunately, the available descriptions and proposed criteria for MCDD seem to be rather over-inclusive and definitely need to be made more specific. However, even with this lack of precision, the available literature suggests that a unique group of individuals is being captured by these criteria. It is important to note that this "group" of individuals are heterogeneous, and may eventually be classified into a number of subgroups or even separate groups.

The symptoms of MCDD can be understood to belong to three major symptom clusters: emotional, cognitive and relational (social). The following list is based on the Towbin, et al. 1993 criteria.

The emotional symptoms betray an impairment in the regulation of affect that goes well beyond the age norms. The intensity, frequency and number of symptoms often suggest multiple coexisting anxiety and/or mood disorders. These symptoms may include: intense generalized anxiety and irritability, recurrent severe panic attacks that are associated with complete disorganization of behavior, multiple unusual phobias that are incapacitating, episodic behavioral disorganization (may not be panic-related) that are extreme and primitive in nature and may include self-injurious behaviors (SIB), a high degree of emotional variability and lability, and/or unusual and incongruent behavioral responses to stress/anxiety-provoking circumstances.

The cognitive symptoms betray an impairment in the processes of thought formation and processing of environmental stimuli. Although these symptoms are somewhat similar to the thought disorders often seen in psychotic disorders, they are usually of a much lesser intensity in MCDD. These symptoms may include: magical thinking inappropriate for age, illogical and bizarre thinking, confusion between reality and fantasy, perplexity and easy confusability, and/or thought systems that approach delusional quality (such as fantasies of omnipotence or grandeur, paranoid ideation, and over-engagement with fantasy figures).

Lastly, the relational/social symptoms betray impairments in social skills, empathy and normal attachment behaviors. The intensity of these deficits lies somewhere between what is observed in PDD and what is common to disruptive behavioral and personality disorders. These symptoms may include: social detachment or superficial attachment that is present in spite of evidence of some capacity for relatedness, inability to initiate or maintain peer relationships, disturbed attachment behaviors toward caregivers (e.g., excessive clinging, aloofness and avoidance, ambivalence, controlling and oppositionality), splitting affects (rapid and easy back and forth shifting between love and hate), and major deficits in empathic skills.

4. Should it be "lumped in" with autism?

Personally, I feel that lumping them with the autism spectrum disorders, which typically means diagnosing them with PDD Not Otherwise Specified (PDDNOS), is not entirely justifiable. Nevertheless, this is the most common approach at present, and it is a reflection of the failure of the current version of the *Diagnostic and Statistical Manual of Mental Disorders* (the DSM-IV-TR) to capture what appears to be a separate diagnostic category. There is no consensus yet about alternatives, but it remains possible to diagnose a subset of these individuals with personality disorders (particularly Schizotypal and Borderline Personality Disorders) and/or psychotic disorders (usually stated as Psychotic Disorder Not Otherwise Specified, and often likened to another unofficial diagnostic term that falls into the psychosis category: Multi-Dimentionally Impaired Disorder or MDI). It might even be argued that MCDD children should be placed in the schizophrenic spectrum, rather than the autistic spectrum, as has previously been proposed for MDI, whose criteria largely overlap those for MCDD.

It may be important to note that when studies have attempted to examine the differences on neurophysiological measures between autism and MCDD, these differences seemed to be rather significant. One illustrative example is the study by Jansen and colleagues (*Neuropsychopharmacology*, 28:582-590, 2003) which showed that MCDD individuals had diametrically opposite physiological responses to stress when compared to autistic individuals.

5. Why don't more doctors and therapists know about this condition?

This is partly because the diagnostic construct is only a proposed one, rather than an official DSM terminology. As such, it will only be well known to some highly specialized child psychiatrists. In addition, this disorder, defined by the Towbin criteria, appears to be rather rare, and the likelihood of clinical experience with this population is rather low. Another factor is that some in the field still use the term "borderline syndrome of childhood," and conceptualize the disorder in a very different manner.

A fourth, and possibly most important factor is that psychiatric training has been influenced very heavily in the past two decades by the DSM system of classification. This leads trainees to be less critical in applying diagnostic criteria. The DSM system is a phenomenologically-based classification system. This means that the diagnostic terms listed in it are descriptors for observable symptom clusters that are agreed upon by the consensus of groups of experts, and may have some supporting epidemiological evidence. However, these disorders are not classified based on underlying neurological correlates. In other words, we believe that these symptoms tend to cluster together, but we don't always know if there is a unifying and shared underlying brain pathology. When there is so much emphasis on the DSM in training and demand for such emphasis by legal, community, industry and systemic interests, these phenomenological descriptors tend to be reified. This leaves less-than-needed room for creative research that may uncover underlying neural correlates of mental illness. MCDD, as a nosological proposal, evolved out of efforts to understand underlying neural and psychological correlates of the pathology observed in children that could not be neatly associated with current DSM diagnostic categories.

It is for these reasons that it would be exceptional for physicians, even for a child psychiatrist, to have substantial knowledge of the MCDD construct.

6. MCDD is not widely known in North America; but seems to be accepted in most other countries. Why do you think this is?

I don't believe that it is accepted in most other countries. It is arguable that there may be more awareness of it in the last decade or so in Europe because some of the seminal research on the disorder was done there. However, the general state of knowledge about MCDD among clinicians is only marginally different, if at all, than it is in North America. The proposed diagnostic criteria for MCDD have not been included in any of the classification systems for mental illness; the two most influential ones are the ICD-10 and the DSM-IV. The ICD-10 is in wider use internationally than the DSM-IV, and the reverse is true in North America. Although it remains unlikely, inclusion of MCDD into an official diagnostic manual is actually more likely to take place in the next iteration of the DSM than it is in the ICD.

7. I have come across many individuals who will not accept the existence of MCDD simply because it has not yet made it into the *Diagnostic and Statistical Manual of Mental Disorders*. In your opinion, what needs to be done to remedy this? How soon do you think this will happen?

As explained in my answer to the 5th question, the DSM has enormous sway on how clinicians think about mental illness. This is neither unusual nor unreasonable. Clinicians are in the business of making diagnoses, and by necessity require a system of classifying conditions. The DSM remains the most legitimate method of reaching diagnoses to the vast majority of clinicians. Despite its many shortcomings, it remains a very useful and currently essential classificatory system. The biggest problem with the DSM, and any classification system for mental illness, is that it will inadvertently reify what remains to be proven real.

The MCDD construct is, to my understanding, likely to be *reviewed* in the process of generating the 5th edition of the DSM. I don't believe it has a big chance of being included in the DSM-V. In the meantime, many children who would otherwise seem to have MCDD could be diagnosed with PDDNOS. The proportion that will now receive this diagnosis has become a bit smaller. This is because of the text revisions introduced in the DSM-IV-TR, which indicated that the diagnosis would apply when impairment in reciprocal social interactions *and* either impaired communication or stereotyped behaviors/interests exist (the DSM-IV, before the *Text Revision*, used the operative *'or'* instead of *'and'*). Others will be diagnosed with either Schizotypal or Borderline Personality Disorder or Psychotic Disorder NOS. Whichever the diagnosis given, it would be unlikely to capture the entire clinical picture, and other diagnoses would probably be assigned, such as Attention-Deficit/Hyperactivity Disorder (ADHD), Oppositional-Defiant Disorder, Generalized Anxiety Disorder, Bipolar Disorder NOS, Panic Disorder, Obsessive-Compulsive Disorder, Learning and Communication Disorders, and even Reactive Attachment Disorder, just to name a few. In my experience, these individuals often have 3-6 DSM diagnoses on Axis I, and may have a few on Axes 2-4. It is definitely not an ideal situation. On the other hand, because of how familiar clinicians are with these other diagnoses, having a child on this multiplicity of diagnoses can give some clinicians an indication of the severity of the condition and intensity of needs of these children and youth.

The only remedy is more research that attempts to further validate the construct and examines the unique therapeutic responses of individuals diagnosed with MCDD. In addition, an in-depth examination of the neural correlates of the disorder and epidemiological studies of its prevalence would greatly improve its chances of being more widely accepted and included in classification systems. Such research is not likely, however, to take place in short order. This is because disorders already identified will tend to attract most of the attention and the research funding necessary.

8. It is unfortunate that past research studies have been flawed. What needs to be done to remedy this situation?

The research that is necessary, not just for MCDD but for all psychiatric diagnoses, is very difficult and time-consuming. The real challenge is to identify the independent components of complex psychiatric symptoms, rather than disorders, that are simple and specific enough to enable detailed neuroscientific study. Once all psychiatric symptoms have undergone such research, and knowledge is accrued about underlying neural correlates, genetic and molecular biological mechanisms, and environmental/psychosocial interactions with this underlying neurobiology, then it may be possible to develop true understanding of the reasons why symptoms may cluster in a specific manner. If such understanding leads us to uncovering a unifying pathology that explains the symptom cluster, we would then have discovered a "disease," rather than simply describing a syndrome or a "disorder," and would then be able to scientifically design studies of therapeutic interventions. In other words, we first need to know what the problem *is*, then we figure out what is causing the problem, then do treatment research based on such understanding.

The above description is a tall order. The current status of research in psychiatry follows the reverse of the above-described path. Presently, we first *agree* that some individuals have a disorder (according to the DSM), then we do treatment research, then results of this research give us reasons to explore how individuals respond, which in turn may tell us something about how the brain works in this group of individuals. This would essentially be a series of research steps that aim to reify what we decided on in the first step, namely that the disorder exists.

This assessment of the current status of psychiatric research is by no means uniquely mine, and is shared by many in the field. However, it would be an unforgivable error to simply dismiss the available research literature as invalid. This research is producing knowledge on an ongoing basis, and improving our ability to help the mentally ill. It is imperfect, but by no means irrelevant.

9. What advice would you give to a parent with a child that has just been diagnosed with MCDD?

Because of the rarity of clinicians that can claim to have specific expertise in diagnosing and treating individuals with MCDD, and because of the relative fluidity of the construct and the remaining uncertainty of it representing a truly unique underlying neuropathology, I would most certainly seek second and even third opinions.

Importantly, I would certainly advise the parent to attempt not to be invested in a *diagnosis* per se. Instead, I would urge them to focus on developing a comprehensive understanding of the child's difficulty with the help of the clinicians. Finding a diagnosis *is not a solution* in the vast majority of cases. A diagnosis is not usually adequate as an explanation, even if it feels that it is, or if it is comforting to believe it is an adequate explanation. In my opinion, a diagnosis helps guide management, but is not an externalizable entity that can be dealt with as an "it."

An assessment of the child needs to ideally include a complete neurodevelopmental evaluation, a complete history of the psychosocial, relational and emotional development of all members of the family and the development of an understanding of what the subjective experience of the child might be. A comprehensive and meaningful explanatory narrative or formulation should result from such an assessment, and aid in developing rationales for treatment.

10. Have there been any brain imaging scans done on children with this condition? If so, how are they different from the scans of children without MCDD?

I am not aware of any brain-imaging studies that have specifically addressed MCDD. However, there have been studies that focused on MDI, comparing it with childhood-onset schizophrenia and normal controls. Given that there is significant overlap between these two proposed diagnostic categories, these studies may prove to be relevant to MCDD. There seem to be significant structural and functional differences between individuals with MDI and those with childhood-onset schizophrenia, but the implications of these differences remain to be examined.

11. What types of therapies and/or treatments do you suggest a patient (with MCDD) have?

Having gone past the diagnostic enquiries, it is important to realize that managing the symptoms of MCDD and addressing the needs of individuals with that diagnosis are not so different than in other severe disorders of childhood. Clinical management must consider that, unlike autism, there may be psychosocial contributions to the onset of the disorder, and there may be a future risk of developing major psychotic disorders or substantial personality pathology.

The focus of any intervention should be improving the quality of life for the child and the family, rather than elimination of symptoms. Reducing or eliminating symptoms may be part of the attempt to improve quality of life, but should not, in my opinion, be the sole goal of treatment. Therefore, treatment should ideally address all of the following:

• Maximizing social and community resources and supports;

• Active and continuing liaison with school staff and any supporting caregivers or mental health workers;

• Full consideration of cultural and religious contexts of the family and the community;

• Individual, family and/or group psychotherapy as indicated;

• Parenting skills, attachment strengthening and behavioral modification interventions as indicated;

• Lifestyle interventions including exercise and dietary modifications; and

• Medications as indicated.

12. What is your opinion of Bettelheim's refrigerator mom theory?

Although there definitely are mothers whose style of parenting could fit the "refrigerator mom" analogy, such styles of parenting do not contribute to the aetiology of autism as was suggested by Bruno Bettelheim. On the other hand, such a style of parenting would in most children contribute to the development of many other psychiatric disorders, but in a much more complex and nuanced manner.

The idea that there could be a simple explanation (or a person to blame) for incredibly complex human behavior, character or relational patterns is basically ludicrous. No matter what disorder we may talk about in psychiatry, there is nearly always a varying degree, depending on the pathology, of interaction between the environment and the genetic/molecular biological make-up of the individual. The environment here refers to everything from the chemical environment within the body, the environment of the womb, birth and early infant-mother interactions, the interplay of child temperament and caregiver character, nutrition and ecological factors, early and late developing relationships, education, to traumatic and significant life events, just to name a few. As for MCDD, it is highly likely that substantial and ongoing gene-environment interactions carry a significant role in both the aetiology and the maintenance of pathology in MCDD.

13. In your opinion, is MCDD a treatable condition?

I don't think the question of *whether* it is a condition has been satisfactorily answered yet. It does seem, however, that many of the symptoms of MCDD can and do improve with comprehensive and complicated treatment regimens, regardless of what the assigned diagnosis is. It is doubtful that all of the symptoms can be eliminated, and there has always been in my experience some residual pathology even in the cases I've had the greatest success with.

14. Is it possible that MCDD could be the result of a disturbing experience for the child; rather than organic in nature? For example, my daughter exhibited symptoms of autism but never aggression until after she started school. She says that she was molested by her special ed teacher. She tells the same story without variation every time she is asked. (I was told by the authorities that her story is unfounded.) It has been three years and she is still afraid to go to school.

This is the sort of question that shows how important it is not to hastily decide that MCDD is a form of PDD, or that it is a form of personality disorder. When people think that it is a form of PDD, there is an assumption that what applies to autism, applies to MCDD. Namely, that it is clearly a developmental disorder that results from powerful genetic factors that begin to influence brain development in utero but peak in their impact in the second year of life, and leave permanent effects on brain function and structure. All of that is just as likely as it unlikely in the case of MCDD.

In fact, there are good reasons to consider a much more prominent impact of the postnatal nurturing and social environment. It turns out that the frequencies of family psychopathology, social adversity and disadvantage, as well as traumatic events are higher in MCDD children than in counterparts that are autistic or have ADHD. It is not yet known whether these factors have *precipitating, perpetuating,* and/or *complicating* effects on the course of the disorder.

As for your daughter, it would be nearly impossible for me based on the snippet of information shared here to be able to either determine the existence of autism or MCDD, or to conclude anything in regards to the possible impact of a traumatic event on her. However, I fully understand why you would be concerned, and I think I would be similarly concerned too. It is obviously important to understand relatively sudden changes in behavior, and difficulties adjusting to specific circumstances or contexts are often among the first things we think about. Sudden change can be caused by discrete experiences or contextual alterations. It is also important to consider the possibility that what appears to be a sudden change may reflect what I call a "threshold phenomenon," where the child lives with a stressor for longer than they can tolerate but only show symptoms when they exhaust their tolerance, or when many small and accumulating stressors accrue beyond the threshold of tolerance. In such circumstances, the appearance of causation could be deceptive.

15. How important is spiritual faith to mental illness?

In my view, it is of great importance. One's faith or spirituality is an essential component of who one is. As such, faith occupies a substantial space in one's subjective reality. Any attempt to address needs that relate to the subjective experience of an individual, such as in mental illness, that does not consider the entirety of the subjective experience is flawed and may be unsuccessful.

16. What is your opinion on taking a holistic approach to treatment? Do you think diet and cleansing of the body helps, or has little or no effect at all?

If you are using the term "holistic" to refer to homeopathic and naturopathic treatments, I would suggest that you consider the following: In my view, *any* treatment has the *potential* of being helpful. Any treatment also has the potential to be harmful. What determines whether a treatment is helpful is evidence generated by research. This applies equally to medical and non-medical interventions. The difference is that, on occasion, the standard of research and the quality of evidence are critiqued differently in medical and non-medical professions. Generally speaking, medical and psychological professions arguably aim for higher-quality evidence. Using such standards of evidence, countless studies have been performed to evaluate whether various common homeopathic and naturopathic interventions could be helpful for psychiatric illnesses. Autism seems to have had the lion share of these studies, none of which established a benefit from the tested homeopathic and naturopathic treatments.

If you are using the term "holistic" to refer to comprehensive treatment that addresses biological, psychological, social, spiritual, cultural, educational, vocational and nutritional facets of individuals with mental illness, then I would most definitely endorse that approach and strongly promote and advocate for it. In fact, that is how I and many in the medical field use that term.

Diet, if it is part of the second definition of "holistic" approach, is a crucial target of intervention. There are dietary modifications that have direct therapeutic or indirect effects, supplant exercise in improving self-esteem, contribute to the management of metabolic effects of some medications, and inculcate a proactively healthy life style. Using diet as a form of "cleansing" intervention would place diet into the former definition of "holistic" approach, and is among the interventions that have failed to produce quality evidence supporting their use in treatment.

17. What do you see the future of mental health to be? Do you think new, improved medications are on the horizon? Better diagnostic testing? A more holistic approach to mental health?

Yes on all three counts, with the caveat that I'm referring to the second definition of the term "holistic," as described in the answer to the previous question.

I believe that with increasing *rapprochement* between clinical observational research, therapeutic research and basic neuroscience research, we will witness an incredible growth in both the knowledge base in psychiatry and the success in managing psychiatric disorder.

18. Is there anything I haven't covered that you would like to add?

I would like to thank you for your efforts to disseminate information to the public about this highly complex, oft confusing subject. I would also like to thank you for inviting me to contribute to those efforts. It is such a complex and multi-faceted issue, that it would be impossible to cover everything in a short interview. However, I do feel that you have touched on most of the important aspects of this issue. Should my responses raise more questions, I would be happy to respond to those as well. Best of luck on this journey of discovery!

Chapter 3

Hello, my name is Jordan. I am going to tell you about my secret hiding place inside my room. Let's take a look at it, shall we? Now, this is my bed, here is my closet. Inside my closet is my secret hiding place. It has two blankets and a great big heart-shaped pillow, and something hanging up top (Bratz lantern) even I have a pirate Scooby Doo. And up on top also I have a hanger who have a nightgown on it and it is a little bit big. Even I have a flashlight, a writing tablet for me. I like my secret hiding place because of I always go in there after school because of it relieves stress out of me. Even I have a flashlight and I am autistic.

—Jordan (on her secret hiding place which she goes to when she is overwhelmed by environmental stimuli)

Naturally, I thought (and sometimes still do think) that Jordan's resistance to attending school stems from the events that happened in the past. In a school meeting (in the county that we now live in) I expressed concerns about this and confessed that Jordan was exhibiting unusual behaviors such as stripping. I said this in an effort to try and make it clear that I believe Jordan has been molested.

Jordan's lack of school attendance turned into truancy charges against me. I went to the court hearing believing that this was the only issue being presented. At the hearing, charges were filed against me for child neglect and abuse. The moral of the story here is to watch what you say (even if you believe it is for the benefit of your child), trust no one, and always have a lawyer to protect the rights of you and your child.

What Causes Autism

If you are a parent who has just learned that their child fits onto the PPD scale, chances are that you are experiencing some degree of guilt. This is not uncommon among parents of handicapped children. Please remember that you did nothing to cause your child's disability. The time you spend feeling guilty is time wasted. It is better for both you and your child that you focus on getting your child the services they need.

While researchers and doctors are still not certain what causes autism; they have a few good ideas. Take solace in the fact that research continues and new discoveries are being made. Recently, genetic research made an amazing discovery which will bring new understanding to the condition, as well as new medication. Here is a summary of what scientists think are potential causes of autism:

Neuro-Immune Dysfunction Syndrome (NIDS)/Autoimmune Disease

In this theory an illness or a vaccine triggers a disease process. The patient would have an immune dysfunction; meaning that their body is not capable of fighting that particular bacteria. As a result, a chemical imbalance is created which causes a restriction in the blood flow in the brain areas controlling speech, language, socialization, and obsessive behaviors.

If this theory holds true, then what is being dealt with is a new type of disease. The good news here is that medications could potentially "cure" autism. Although this theory has not yet been proven, research patients are showing amazing improvements upon being treated.

MMR Vaccines

One of the most promising research studies is that of MMR (measles, mumps, and rubella) vaccines. Researchers have found measles in the gastrointestinal tract of autistic children. There are reports of children who could talk and were socially active until after they received the MMR vaccine. They became reclusive and stopped talking within a week of receiving it.

Despite what would seem an obvious link, the federal government has not yet recognized the need to change its standards on vaccines. Because of this, the MMR vaccine is still required for entry into the public school system. A person concerned with the MMR vaccine may get out of this requirement by having a letter from a clergy person saying that it is against religious beliefs. A doctor may also write a letter saying that the vaccine is harmful to your child's health. If both of these ideas fail, you may want to consider homeschooling your children.

Mercury

Waters in the United States are currently so polluted that the FDA has put a warning on eating fish. This is because of the large amounts of a metal called mercury that is in our waterways. Mercury has already been proven as a link in birth defects; so much so that pregnant women are advised not to eat any fish. In this theory, children on the PDD scale have an unusually large amount of mercury in their bodies.

There are promising research studies being conducted in this area. In these studies, children are put through a cleansing process to rid the body of mercury. Children who receive this treatment have also shown improvement.

Genetics

The most recent discovery on autism is also the most exciting and definitive to date. Researchers have pinpointed a gene (called MET) variant that more than doubles the chances of a child being born autistic.

The MET gene is active in the brain both before and after birth. MET helps support brain functions in the regions that control language, emotion, digestion, and the immune system.

This opens up for further research into the vaccine and mercury connection. Up until now there has not been any hard scientific evidence to support these theories. Now, researchers are hoping to find a connection with the MET gene. The theory is that the MET variant makes people highly sensitive to vaccines and mercury, thus contributing to the effects of autism.

The discovery of this gene variant also opens up doors for new ways to treat autism. Researchers are hoping to find a way to boost the MET gene, and therefore lessen the effects of autism.

Silicon

In California, the area where computers are made (dubbed Silicon Valley) has seen an ever-increasing rise in the number of new cases of autism. In Silicon Valley there are seven new cases reported every day.

Chapter 4

*Sometimes my dreams scare me because I have to run away
from my fear. And then I get brave and courage. Even then I go
face my fears. Even I always sometimes get afraid of my dreams.
That is why I always run away from the fears that I get. Sometimes
my brains think all of the confusion and it makes scary things.
Some dreams are good, some dreams are bad, some dreams are
scary. But, you always have to remember to face your fears. Even
one time I had a dream that was so scary that I had to run away
from the monster. And then I faced my fears. You always have to
face your fears. And, my name is Jordan Clemons and this story
is not over.*

—Jordan talking about her dreams

It was a morning that I will never forget. The wind was blowing
fiercely and there was a silence in the air (the kind that only comes with
winter's chill). Things had come to a head with the school system. I
knew that something was wrong with my child but I didn't know what.

The worst part was that nobody at her school would listen to me. When they did, I received answers that fit the typical child. These answers did not fit my child nor did they ease my worries.

I was being told that Jordan was just experiencing difficulties adjusting to the school routine. The answer, I was told, was to be more firm. I was told straight out that Jordan's lack of school attendance was becoming a problem and that criminal charges would be filed against me.

I had been trying, unsuccessfully, to get Jordan to school that morning. The day started with Jordan running out of the house and down the street totally naked. After about 20 minutes of chasing her through our neighborhood, I had finally coaxed her into the house. I got her dressed and into the car. We were less than a mile from school when Jordan undid her seat belt, climbed over the front seat of the car, opened the car door and attempted to jump out. My reaction was to let go of the steering wheel and grab the back of my daughter's shirt. I kept her in the car but in the process almost hit the car in the lane next to me.

Once at school, Jordan managed to wedge herself underneath the gas pedal of my car. Luckily, there happened to be an emergency response team at the school (there for a demonstration). The response team managed to get Jordan out of my car. She latched on to me and sunk her teeth into my neck. The school responded by calling the department of mental health. A worker came to the school and tried to convince me to have my daughter detained in a mental hospital. Jordan has always had a fear of separation and I had promised her several times that I would never leave her. I felt that (by having her committed) she would perceive it as my breaking that promise. I felt that the separation anxiety issue would just be made worse. I stood firm in my refusal. We finally reached a compromise. I would allow a private social worker to come into my home. I also agreed for my daughter to be seen and diagnosed (as an outpatient) by the mental health department.

After only one 20-minute visit at the mental health department, my daughter was diagnosed with separation anxiety. I was told that all she needed was an antidepressant and to be forced to go to school. The mental health department then wrote my daughter a prescription for a pill that she could not swallow. Their advice resulted in Jordan breaking my nose one morning on the way to school. The next morning her social worker attempted to take her to school. Jordan kicked her in the face.

Now I know that Jordan's behavior was partly due to her inability to cope with the overwhelming amount of environmental stimulation at school. The school environment was physically painful to her and she could not communicate this to anyone. In desperation she was attempting to run away from the cause of the pain (in her case school). She simply could not cope with the fluorescent lighting, the loud sounds made by other children, nor could she process her way around the school building.

Imagine if you were locked in a world where the most ordinary things in life caused you great distress, even physical pain. Imagine that you could not tell anyone. Imagine that those whom you trusted the most, the very ones that were supposed to protect you, were forcing you into those situations of stress. When you think like this; Jordan's actions start to make sense.

What Behaviors to Expect from an Autistic Child:

Meltdowns: A meltdown can be described as a temper tantrum that escalates, but unlike a temper tantrum, the autistic child cannot calm themselves down. Meltdowns can last from minutes to hours. Meltdowns can include cursing, hitting, yelling, biting, and kicking. Most often, meltdowns are caused by an exterior stimulant. In Jordan's case, she cannot handle the lighting in most department stores. When she is with me, I must limit my shopping to 40 minutes. To extend our trip beyond this point usually results in Jordan cursing, hissing at strangers, kicking me, and acting like a horse (complete with neighing and galloping).

Cursing: It is not unusual for children on the PPD spectrum to have Tourette's syndrome. With Tourette's a person experiences uncontrollable periods of cursing. If your child has Tourette's it is imperative that you remember that cursing is a symptom of a disease and not something that should be punished. While your child's episodes may be improved with medication and behavior therapy, your child is not willingly in control of their cursing. In short, it's not their fault.

Crying: Crying often and for long periods of time is the PPD child's way of communicating frustration or need. Remember an autistic child has different priorities than the rest of us. Jordan's Littlest Petshop toys must be lined up just right. She notices if one has been moved just the tiniest bit. I have practically given up trying to dust this area of her room. If I accidentally move one out of place, Jordan will notice. The result is her crying and throwing objects across the room.

Obsessive Compulsive Behaviors: Although annoying to the rest of us, these behaviors are something that your child is not choosing to be obsessed with; they just are. Possible compulsive disorders to look for: lining up objects, opening and closing doors, spinning in a circle, hand or arm flapping, rocking back and forth, counting objects repeatedly for no particular reason, hiding objects, and objects must always be placed in a certain location.

Elopement: The autistic child often feels the need to get away from it all. They do this by running away (called elopement). Jordan will do this whenever she is upset. For her, it is even more dangerous because she takes off her clothes during the process. I suggest that parents and caregivers install alarm systems. Most good systems announce when a door opens and which door it is. In this way you can keep an ear out for your child attempting to leave the house without you. Another plus, you will know if your child sneaks out at night because the alarm will wake you up.

What Behaviors to Expect from a Child with MCDD

Children with MCDD display the same set of behaviors as the PDD child, with some additional ones.

Inability to differentiate between fantasy and reality: MCDD children can get caught up in their fantasy world to the point that they start to believe in it. And no amount of persuasion from adults can make them believe otherwise. Jordan loves dragons and she continually asks what her guardian dragon is doing. If you child comes up with a farfetched tale, don't punish them for fibbing. It is important to remember that in your child's mind these things are real. Be patient and remember that this is a symptom beyond your child's immediate control.

Unusual attachment to a caregiver that can quickly turn violent: Jordan can be hugging me one moment and then strangling me the next. Research suggests that children take out their anger where they feel the safest—usually a loved one.

Unusual fears: Unusual fears manifest themselves in some very odd ways. What an average child or adult may fear, an MCDD child may not. At the same time, ordinary things that the rest of us take for granted can cause stress. Jordan loves roller coasters, and the faster and more extreme—the more she likes them. She can't wait until she is tall enough to get on the Volcano. The Volcano is an extreme roller coaster that shoots the rider out of the top of a flaming volcano. Every few weeks Jordan measures herself to see if she is tall enough. She is tall enough to get on the Anaconda. This is a roller coaster which goes upside down and has corkscrews. Just the very thought of the Anaconda makes my heart start beating faster. I will even break out in a sweat. Jordan loves it and she will ride it over and over again if she is allowed to. On the other hand, the sight of Elmer's glue sends her screaming and running into another room.

Intense anxiety and anger: The MCDD child has intense anxiety which can quickly turn to anger and violence. In Dutch studies questioning the child about their anger seems to only make them more aggressive. Dutch studies have shown that children with MCDD seem to become stronger during periods of high anxiety, which can be compared to the effect that LSD has on the body.

Psychotic thinking: Children with MCDD have reported hearing voices in their heads. They can also become paranoid and think that the whole world is against them or that people are talking about them.

Uncontrolled aggression: Children with MCDD often say that they are aware of their aggressive behaviors but that they cannot gain control over their actions.

Fear which easily leads to fury: It is believed that the extreme anger and aggression exhibited by children with MCDD may actually be a reaction to fear. Researchers believe that environmental stimuli is the cause of fear which leads to fury.

Frustration over what they know they can do and what their disability limits them to doing. Jordan has an average IQ, however, she has difficulty with language skills. She wants to learn to read and she knows that she can do it, but her inability to control her emotions interferes with her ability to stay on task. This results in frustration, which leads to anger, which leads to her injuring me when she gets home from school.

Eating problems: Jordan does not recognize when she is full and will eat up to three or four plates of food at dinner if allowed to.

Sleep problems: Children with MCDD experience great difficulty with falling to sleep and then sleeping through the night.

Behavior Strategies to Try:

I have had the help of a very good (privately employed) social worker towards improving Jordan's behaviors. Here is a list of some things that have worked for us.

Communication board: Although this is a piece of assistive technology; we have used it very successfully towards decreasing the amount of meltdowns. We believe this is because, with the help of the communication board, Jordan is able to effectively communicate her needs.

Emotions communication board: Again, this can be considered assistive technology, however, it helps reduce meltdowns by enabling your child to express his/her feelings before they reach meltdown level.

A schedule chart: Children on the PDD scale need a daily routine. Researchers suspect that this gives the PDD child a sense of security because they know what to expect next. Chances are that your family has some type of routine and you may not even be aware of it. What time does your family wake up in the morning? What time is bedtime? What about chores and homework? All of this information can easily be turned into a calendar. Hang the calendar where your autistic child can easily see it and reach it. Each day go through your daily routine while checking things on the calendar. For example, when you first get up, have your child move the check mark or other marker to the wake up slot on the calendar. Then your child will move the marker to school time. When they get home from school, the marker will be moved to homework, then down time, etc.

Directions for making a schedule chart:

Materials:

Glue
Photos representing daily activities (clip art can also be used)
Felt
Velcro
Scissors
Markers
A ruler
Poster board

Instructions:

Pick out photos or clip art to represent your child's daily activities. For example, a clip art of a plate of food can represent dinner. Or, you could take an actual photo of your child eating dinner.

Using a marker, section off the poster board into four vertical sections and eleven horizontal sections. The horizontal sections each represent daily activities such as wake up, go to school, homework, brush teeth, etc. The vertical sections are for time, activity name in words, the activity picture, and a place for a marker.

Cut the photos down to the size that you want.

Start at the top with "waking up" and work your way down to "bedtime." Glue a photo in the third column of each row.

The first column is to be left blank. This is where the marker will go.

In the second column write in the time of the day in which the activity takes place.

The third column should already be finished with the photos.

In the fourth column write the activity name in words.

Decide what your will use as a marker. For Jordan's schedule, we used art work of a dragon which we got off the net.

Cut the marker photo down to size. Glue the photo to the back of a piece of felt that has been cut down to the same size as the photos. Glue a small piece of felt to the back of the marker.

Glue a small piece of felt to each row of the first column.

Teach your child to move the marker at the beginning of each daily activity.

An example of a daily schedule

A secret hiding place: Jordan has a secret hiding place where she can go when she becomes overwhelmed. The secret hiding place has been successful in our fight against elopement. Now, instead of running down the street naked, Jordan removes her clothes inside her secret hiding place. Jordan's secret hiding place is her closet. We removed the bars used for hanging clothes, shoe racks, etc., from her closet. We then decorated it by hanging a lantern from the ceiling. The floor is covered with blankets and pillows. We added a flashlight, books, and markers for Jordan to enjoy.

You do not have to use a closet. A pop-up tent, a tree house, etc., can also be used to create a secret hiding place. Remember, the secret hiding place is somewhere your child can go when they feel overwhelmed. It is never to be used as time out or any other form of punishment.

Positive reinforcement: Research studies have shown that positive reinforcement is the best behavior management therapy for children with autism. It can be easily done and it does not have to be costly. First, pinpoint the behaviors you want your child to improve on. Try to word your behaviors in positive ways. One of Jordan's goals is to always wear shoes when she goes outdoors. We could say, "Jordan needs to stop going outside barefooted." But, instead we say, "Jordan gets a sticker every time she wears shoes outside." Make a calendar that your child can place stickers on. (This calendar does not have to be anything elaborate. We use our yearly calendar. Since the target behaviors are limited, Jordan is capable of keeping track of what the stickers are for.) Jordan gets to pick something out of the goody bag every time she earns five stickers. The goody bag is filled with candy and things brought at our local dollar store. At the end of the month, if she earns all of her stickers, she gets to go out to the movies.

It is important that you only work at one or two behaviors at a time. The goal is to help your child to feel positive about themselves. You want to set up the positive reinforcement program in a way in which your child cannot fail.

Meltdowns: Meltdowns are more easily avoided than they are fixed. The best advice is to figure out what causes a meltdown and then try to avoid them. It helps Jordan to take her Game Boy with her when we go out. She concentrates more on the game and less on the external stimuli around her.

Back off: Oftentimes, attempts at controlling an MCDD child's behavior will backfire, resulting in increased anxiety and aggression. If you are attempting to intervene in your child's behavior and the behavior seems to be increasing as a result, it may be best to just back off for a few moments.

Use clear and concise language: When speaking with your

child, use short sentences instead of long, drawn-out ones. When you want your child to do something, use commands containing as few a words as possible. For example, instead of saying, "It is now time to go to bed," simply say, "Go to bed." Speak slowly to give your child time to process the information.

Lower the speed at which a task should be done: It is important to allow autistic and MCDD children more time to complete tasks. You should provide them frequent breaks and entertainment choices during these breaks.

Keep the focus on the perception of the child: You will be able to understand your child much better resulting in much more effective behavior strategies if you constantly strive to see things through the perception of your child.

Plan ahead: When planning an outing or a family gathering, know ahead of time about the number of people who will be there, the type of lighting, etc. Plan a behavior strategy ahead of time which includes meltdowns, escape plans, etc.

Be creative with your behavior therapies: (For example, Jordan does not like to wear underwear because they are tight fitting. We solved this by buying her boy's boxers.) And remember, behaviors do not change overnight. It takes a great deal of effort and dedication on everyone's part in order for any behavior program to be successful.

If you find that your child's negative behaviors are increasing; then something is wrong. Take a deep breath, step back, and investigate what is wrong in your child's life. It may not be your behavior program. It is possible that the problem may be in school, on the playground, or with a sibling. Remember that children with MCDD will withhold information about a problem. It is not that they withhold the information to be in control of you, but because they lack the capacity to communicate the situation to you. Negative behaviors are usually a result of your child's frustration at a problem.

Chapter 5

When I grow up I know that I have two things that I want to do when I grow up. I want to work at home. Even I want to be a horses back rider and get money from it. Even, I like to run for President of the United States. 'Cause of I don't know how to be a President, that's why I want to be one. I would change that there would be video games and more money for poor people, even rich people. I would make food and doctors. Even shelter for the animals. And, I will have shelter for any type of animal. Even doctors for humans. And that is it.

—Jordan (on what she wants to do when she grows up)

The poor service we received at our mental health department made me determined to do things my way. I requested that Jordan's primary doctor refer Jordan to a local hospital that specialized in children. There, Jordan received (what I thought was) a thorough evaluation. After three hours of questions and observations, I received a two-page report that basically said nothing. There was one sentence that mentioned PDD. There was no explanation about the meaning of it (the term autism was never used in the report). There was no reference to follow-up visits nor was my daughter referred to any types of therapies (i.e.: behavioral, occupational, etc.). Jordan did receive speech therapy for one year at this same facility.

The social worker had stopped visiting Jordan (due to health insurance issues) and I was looking for a child psychologist. I saw an ad in our phone book for equine therapy. Knowing Jordan's love for horses, I could think of nothing that would be better for her. Luckily, the equine therapist was also a child psychologist with a clue about autism. The former director of a children's mental health hospital, he quickly recognized Jordan's symptoms.

He read through the two previous evaluations that had been done on Jordan. He said that the mental health facility had totally missed the mark. The evaluation from the children's facility was quickly written and said "a lot of nothing." Words cannot describe the elation I felt upon hearing this. Finally, someone who understood!

He referred Jordan to our city's university health center. There Jordan was evaluated and it was determined that Jordan does not just have autism, but multiple complex developmental disorder. Finally, real answers that made sense to me.

What to Look for in a Physician

Getting the best physicians for your child is going to take a lot of research. Don't just assume that (because the doctor has a degree) every doctor has the means to give your child a proper diagnosis. Getting a proper diagnosis of MCDD is extremely hard for several reasons: because it is not a common known condition in the United States; because the MCDD child is able to function and communicate well; and their incapacity to withstand stimuli is often misunderstood as an unwillingness to cooperate. While getting a proper diagnosis is hard, it is not impossible. Here are a few pointers that may help:

Research: Look on the web for information regarding your child's potential physician. Are they up on the latest research? Have they won any awards or praise from the community or other doctors? Where did they go to college? (Research the school the doctor graduated from). Have they done any research on your child's health condition? Have they published any papers?

Research the facility the doctor is affiliated with: Does the facility have a good record? Have there ever been any accusations of abuse or health code violations? Does the facility have a reputation for using a lot of medication? Has the facility conducted or participated in any recent research? Are the staff friendly? Do they take an interest in your child?

Interview: If possible, schedule an interview with the doctor before your child's first visit. (Caution: You may have to pay out of pocket for this, but it's worth it.) The most important aspect of the interview is to see whether or not you have a rapport with the doctor. Does the doctor listen to your concerns? Does the doctor value your opinion? Does the doctor take the time that is necessary to explain things to you and answer your questions? What is the doctor's attitude concerning medications? What is their attitude towards natural health and alternative medicines? Does the doctor have contacts with other services that he/she can refer you to? How much experience does the doctor have working with children on the autism spectrum? (Note: It is relatively easy to diagnose an autistic child who has all of the classic symptoms. If your child is high functioning you will want to look for someone who has had experience working with children who have Asperger's).

Try to stay away from public health facilities (i.e. your county's local health department): I am sure that this is a controversial statement that I am going to get a great deal of flak for saying. However, I have found it to be true. I am not saying that county health departments do not have qualified doctors. But, for whatever reason, I have found that they do not make good diagnoses. Take into consideration that your local health department is working on a tight budget. The doctor there is more than likely not getting paid the same as if they were in private practice. They are trying to see as many people as they can within the shortest amount of time possible. (This is not to say that they don't want to do their job. This is because there are so many people needing services). If you have no choice but to use the mental health facility, then do so but be firm in your opinions and what you want for your child. It may take more than one visit to get what you want. If your child has typical symptoms your fight will probably not be as difficult as the person whose child has PPD with MCDD.

Sometimes you may have to go out of plan: You may find that your insurance plan does not have a doctor which you find suitable. In these cases, it may be necessary to go out of your plan. In some cases, this may mean paying out of pocket. Again, it is worth spending the cash in order to get your child's diagnosis. Check beforehand to see if you can make payment arrangements with the doctor. You may need to use this out-of-plan doctor only to get a proper diagnosis for your child. Once your child is diagnosed, you can again use an in-plan doctor for follow-up treatments and services.

The DSM-IV Criteria for Autistic Disorder

This is what most physicians use to determine if a child meets the criteria for autism. A child must have at least six of the twelve symptoms listed. Your child meets the criteria for having a specific symptom if they exhibit one or more of the behaviors associated with that symptom. Of the symptoms listed, your child must exhibit at least two of the behaviors listed under reciprocal social intervention, at least one symptom under communication, and one symptom under restricted repetitive behaviors.

DSM-IV Criteria for Autistic Disorder

Deficits in reciprocal social interaction
1a. Difficulty using nonverbal behaviors to regulate social interaction.
• Trouble looking others in the eye

• Little use of gestures while speaking
• Few or unusual facial expressions
• Trouble knowing how close to stand to others
• Unusual intonation or voice quality

1b. Failure to develop age-appropriate peer relationships.
• Few or no friends
• Relationships only with those much older or younger than the child or with family members.
• Relationships based primarily on special interests
• Trouble interacting in groups and following cooperative rules of games

1c. Little sharing of pleasure, achievements, or interests with others
• Enjoys favorite activities, television shows, toys alone, without trying to involve other people
• Does not try to call others' attention to activities, interests, or accomplishments
• Little interest in, or reaction to praise

1d. Lack of social or emotional reciprocity.
• Does not respond to others, appears deaf
• Not aware of others, oblivious to their existence
• Strongly prefers solitary activities
• Does not notice when others are hurt or upset; does not offer comfort
• Deficits in communication

2a. Delay in or total lack of development of language.
• No use of words to communicate by age two
• No simple phrases (for example, "more milk") by age three
• After speech develops, immature grammar or repeated errors

2b. Difficulty building conversations.

• Has trouble knowing how to start, keep going, and/or end a conversation
• Little back and forth; may talk on and on in a monologue
• Fails to respond to the comments of others, responds only to direct questions
• Difficulty talking about topics not of special interest

2c. Unusual or repetitive language.
• Repeating what others say to them
• Repeating from videos, books, or commercials at inappropriate times or out of context
• Using special words or phrases that have been made up or have special meaning only to the child
• Overly formal style of speaking

2d. Play that is not appropriate for developmental level.
• Little acting out scenarios with toys
• Rarely pretends that an object is something else (example: an empty box is a house or a car)
• Prefers to use toys in a concrete manner other than playing pretend with them
• Little interest in social games such as peek a boo and ring around the rosie
• Restrictive, repetitive behaviors, interests or activities

3a. Interests that are narrow in focus, overly intense, and/or unusual.
• Very strong focus on particular topics to the exclusion of other topics
• Difficulty letting go of special topics or activities
• Interference with other activities
• Interest in topics that are unusual for age (for example—Jordan loves to go on extreme roller coasters that go upside down and do spiral twists)
• Excellent memory for details of special interest

3b. Unreasonable insistence on sameness and following familiar routines.
• Wants to perform certain activities in an exact order (for example, close all doors in a specific order)
• Easily upset about minor changes in routine
• Need for advanced warning of any changes
• Becomes highly anxious and upset if routines or rituals not followed

3c. Repetitive motor mannerisms
• Flapping hands when excited or upset
• Flicking fingers in front of eyes
• Odd hand postures or other hand movements
• Spinning or rocking for long periods of time
• Walking and/or running on tiptoe

3d. Preoccupation with parts of objects
• Uses objects in unusual ways
• Interest in sensory qualities of objects (Jordan must smell her feet after removing her shoes and socks)
• Likes objects that move or spin
• Attachment to unusual objects

The Huge Scary Dog Who Is Nice
(by Jordan Clemons)

Half wolf and half coyote
That dog was huge
It chases after the little dog that I like
I really do like that little dog
That coyote wolf chases after him
The little dog knows that the wolf dog won't hurt him
That wolf dog got run over by a tractor
Now he has bolts and screws inside his back leg
Now he needs to take it slowly when he gets up
It turns out that that coyote wolf was really nice

Chapter 6

Hello, I just told a mommy who just found out that their kid have autism. This is the first thing if they have the autism where they can talk (that is me) then be aware of fighting, kicking, screaming, even stronger than you, and biting. Even you need to protect them from your head, your hair, your face. Even if they have where they can't talk they will pinch and kick and grab and scream. Even there is another one who can't talk either. When they see their mom they will think they have to go home. Even he hit his head. Even calm them down. Even help them to talk and write. Make a happy face. And be aware of what they want can talk. If they run outside naked or run away. I don't know they can like calm down, breathe, say I still love you. In case they think their mom don't love them at all. Calm down. Say I still love your. Say don't run away. Give them popsicles, give them video games. Even give them what they want but that will take some while but that will come true, right? And, remember, always be good.

—Jordan (advice to parents)

I hired a lawyer to protect my rights and to represent me in the court proceedings. The hearing was postponed while my lawyer prepared our case. Meanwhile, I received a bill in the mail (from the court) for the amount of $529. I asked my lawyer what the charges were for. His assistant called the court and was told that the charges were for court fees and state attorney's fees. Charges which we felt I should not have to pay since the hearings had not yet been held. She was told that I had to pay only $89 now and the rest after the hearing.

The court date arrived and we were told by the judge that he would not proceed because I had not paid the court fees. We explained what the clerk told us. The hearing was postponed another 60 days—meanwhile I was to pay the full amount.

A few weeks later I went to the clerk's office to pay the fees. It was lunchtime, the line of people went out the door and there was only one person working the window. I was told by this person that I had paid my fines in full. I explained that the judge demanded that I pay the $529. The clerk said that I had to be mistaken because there were no outstanding fees. I then asked her for a printout with her name on it; which showed that I owed nothing. She grumbled and then said she would pull my file. Several minutes later she returned and said that their computer system had different information than that which was in my file. I was to pay the full amount.

The clerk's office refunded my money to me a week before the court date. Another lesson learned—keep your sense of humor or you will go insane.

Medicating Your Child

Whether or not to medicate your child is a personal decision. Only you can decide whether or not your child's symptoms are so severe that medication is necessary. Remember that all medication comes with side effects. Children are being medicated at an alarmingly young age (some as early as five). The long-term effects of most medications have not yet been determined. It is important to keep in mind that medication will only address the symptoms associated with PDD's, and will not address the core symptoms (such as not talking, etc.).

Alternative Medicines

Alternative medicine has grown in popularity. No longer the choice of just tree huggers, modern scientific research has found evidence that many ancient herbs and remedies really do work. Even The National Institute of Health (NIH) is currently conducting research on the effect acupuncture has on autism.

If you decide to go this route I highly recommend that you do so under the supervision of a qualified naturopathic doctor or herbal practitioner. You will be using only natural substances but you should keep in mind that herbs and vitamins can cause allergic reactions and may build up toxic levels in the body.

Finding a Qualified Naturopathic Practitioner

You will want to locate a qualified herbal practitioner or naturopathic doctor; one that holds a degree in the field. Here are the four types of degrees to look for:

Naturopathic Doctor: (ND) To qualify for this degree the practitioner must have studied for four years at an accredited naturopathic medical school.

MNIMH or FNIMH: This degree is obtained by study at the National Institute for Medical Herbalism in England.

American Herbalist Guild (AHG): Members certified by the AHG are reviewed by a panel, and must have completed the equivalent of three to four years of training.

Licensed Acupuncturist (LA): To earn this license an acupuncturist must have completed an extensive training program.

Possible Causes of Autism and How They Can Be Treated Naturally

In a previous chapter I covered what researchers think may cause autism. Natural medicine provides relatively cheap ways to treat these.

Mercury: Naturopathic doctors say that clay removes mercury and other metals from the body. Good clay bath products are available for this. Who knew that making mud pies could be good for your health? Other natural ways to cleanse mercury from the body include: cilantro, vitamin C, garlic, and Vitamin E.

Brain functions: Researchers at Harvard are now studying the use of fish oil and omega three fatty acids in the treatment of depression and bipolar disorder. Omega three fatty acids support proper brain function.

Acupuncture: It is believed that acupuncture stimulates the liver and kidneys, thus flushing the body from mercury and other toxins.

Herbal Treatments for Common PDD Symptoms

Many symptoms which are now being treated with prescription medications can also be treated with herbs. Following is a list of common symptoms and the herbs that are used to treat them. Herbal teas can usually be drunk once every two hours. Follow manufacturer's suggestions for tablets. Or, better still, follow your practitioner's advice.

Anxiety: Chamomile, linden, vervain, motherwort, St. John's wort, hops, skullcap, kava-kava, valerian, passionflower, Siberian ginseng, licorice, lavender oil (not to be taken internally).

Depression: Oats, lavender (external only), vervain, ginkgo, kava-kava.

Sleeplessness: Valerian, California poppy, lemon balm, passionflower, kava-kava, chamomile, skullcap, catnip.

Obsessive-Compulsive Disorder: St. John's wort, kava-kava, valerian, California poppy, bergamot (external use).

Chapter 7

I don't like school because of I don't have time to write in my writing tablet anymore. Even, it is about to drive me insane and crazy. And it is about to make me mad. I don't want to do homework anymore. Even, less work. Even, I don't like to work that much any more. And I am about to bite my mom and go insane. Homework is going to make me do the same thing too. And, if anybody comes to bother me I am going to hit them inside the f__king balls and inside the f__king face. And crazy! And the classroom is driving me crazy, too. The lights—I thought that they were supposed to calm me down. But they don't at all.

More time to write on my writing tablet. Even little lights, if they can make it. Even, less homework and less work. Even I want to have less work time anywhere. More exercise and that is it.

—Jordan (having a bad day at school)

Jordan loves horses. Equine therapy is one of the best ways I have found for Jordan to relax. We noted a difference in Jordan's behavior after just a few sessions with an equine therapist. Her self-confidence was boosted. She started to come out of her own little world and into ours. Her mood is always much more relaxed for a few days after she goes riding.

She has graduated from equine therapy to regular horseback riding lessons. She just started this and she loves it. Her behavior program has been expanded so that she can now earn bigger prizes such as riding helmets, riding boots, etc.

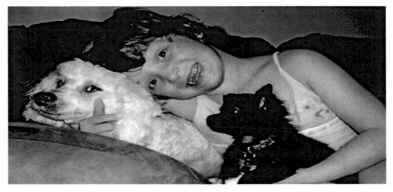

Dogs can serve several purposes: they provide companionship, a sense of security, and teach responsibility.

Therapy

If you have a child on the PPD or MCDD spectrum, you will want to provide him/her with every opportunity for growth. I find that the most successful for Jordan has been a combination of animal therapies and organized sports activities.

Animal Therapy: Animals provide a safe haven for a child. Animals are forgiving, they do not judge, and they are accepting of your child with all of his/her disabilities. A dog can be your child's best friend.

Service Dogs: Service dogs are an excellent choice. Not only will a service dog be your child's best friend, but it will also provide you with some peace of mind. Service dogs are trained to do several things including: protecting your child from strangers, find its way home if your child becomes lost, and assist your child in everyday activities.

Equine Therapy: Equine therapy or horseback riding provides children with a sense of accomplishment, what it is like to have something to care for and, it soothes the mind, body, and soul.

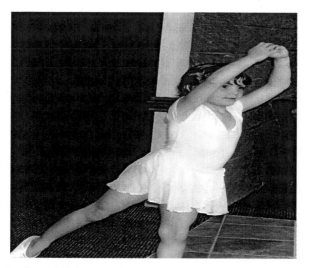

Organized activities such as ballet provide opportunities for social interaction, a sense of accomplishment, and improve fine motor skills.

Organized Sports: Organized sporting events such as soccer, softball, and track and field are wonderful ways for your child to boost self-confidence while improving balance and motion skills. You do not have to go out and join the YMCA or sign up for your local league. Your local Special Olympics chapter can provide a list of free activities that your child can participate in. It is also good for you, the parent, because you will meet other parents who are facing the same difficulties and life choices.

Private Social Workers: Private social workers usually have degrees in psychology and/or education. They are specially trained to know what services are available in the community and how to go about applying for them. Jordan's social worker has been invaluable by providing behavior strategies and working with the schools.

Child Psychologists: Child psychologists can also work with your child on self-esteem issues and behavior problems. A good psychologist is someone you want in your corner when dealing with the school system.

Cognitive Behavior Therapy: Dutch researchers report excellent results using Cognitive Behavior Therapy to treat children with MCDD. In this technique children are taught how to replace negative thoughts and actions with positive ones.

ABA Therapy: The only scientifically proven method to treat autism symptoms is ABA (Applied Behavioral Analysis) therapy. This type of therapy involves an extensive amount of time (30 to 40 hours a week) under the supervision of a trained therapist. With ABA therapy an autistic child learns daily tasks in a one-step-at-a-time approach. For example: when learning to brush their teeth, the autistic child will first learn to pick up their toothbrush and toothpaste. After they have mastered this they will learn to unscrew the toothpaste cap. Positive reinforcement is used throughout the program as a way to award each new task learned.

Sensory Integration Therapy: Sensory integration therapy is used to help the child cope with the overwhelming amount of external stimuli in their everyday environment. Sensory integration therapy involves putting the child into a room filled with environmental stimuli. Fun activities are planned to try and help the child learn to better cope with stimuli.

Art Therapy: It is believed that the creative process of making visual arts is in itself healing and life enhancing. A professional art therapist is trained to pick up on subtle hints in the child's art work that may be clues to issues that need to be dealt with.

Music Therapy: A therapist uses music as a means to improve motor skills, social/interpersonal development, cognitive development, self-awareness, and spiritual enhancement.

Assistive Technologies

Communication Boards: Communication boards serve several functions. Not only do they allow your child a means to communicate their needs but, by doing so your child may decrease the number of meltdowns. Communication boards do not have to be expensive pieces of technology. You can make one at home with a few craft supplies: poster board, glue, pictures and clip art printed off the computer. Simply pick out photos and clip art that represent different needs your child may have: tired, sick, toileting, hungry, etc. Also have some safety information on the communication board such as name, address, and the words "I'm lost" or "I need help." Simply glue the photos and information onto a board which has been cut down to a convenient size. Teach your child to point to the different pictures to express their needs.

Emotions Board: An emotions board is very similar to a communications board. Only, instead of needs, find photos or clip art which represent different emotions: happy, sad, angry, hurt, etc. Jordan's communication board also includes different activities she can choose to relieve stress, such as: secret hiding place, bike riding, etc.

Sign Language: Sign language is another way to help your child to communicate. One drawback with sign language is that everyone in your child's life will need to learn it with him/her. Others in the community probably will not know it and, therefore, not be able to understand what your child is trying to say.

Occupational Therapy: Occupational therapy helps your child with the skills needed for everyday survival (i.e. brushing their teeth, using a fork, etc). A wide variety of tools are available to occupational therapists. Your child may be given specially shaped forks, a motorized wheelchair or even a computer.

One of the things that an occupational therapist may work on with your child is sensory integration. Sensory integration exercises are designed to help the autistic child to become less sensitive to the environment around them.

Speech Therapy: Speech therapy is designed to encourage the autistic child to make sounds which could lead to speech. A child that can speak will be trained to improve their sounds so that others might be able to understand them.

Chapter 8

I know something about bees. All right, inside flower, and like, trees, leaves. Inside there they have pollen and that is how bees make the, the honey. And like, if you smack on them, then they will think that you will fight them. There is a kind of bee where they are in a whole pack and coming at you at the same time. Then you have to go in the house. Normal bees, um, just don't smack at them. Just stay still and don't move. Then they won't mind you or bother you. Now, there is a lot of honey bees. And, this one time, um, when me and my mom were outside there were bees all over our plum tree. And the other time when we were at the park there was a sweat bee and this little girl and this little boy run away. Even then, I told them that if you run away if you go like this (smacks with hands) even then they will sting you. And butterflies come out of worms. And that is it.

—Jordan (on bees and butterflies)

I was told that the only way the county would provide Jordan with the educational setting she needs is if I gave up custody of her. I sat stunned and in disbelief. To rub salt in my wounds, this news was coming from Jordan's lawyer; the person on our side. Jordan's doctors say that she needs to attend a special day program (during normal school hours). There she would receive not just an education but be evaluated for possible medications. She would receive speech and occupational therapies. Jordan would be under the care of a qualified team of psychologists who would work with me to improve her behaviors. Unfortunately, this program is not covered by medical insurance and comes with the costly price tag of $40,000 a year. Since it is considered an alternative school setting, the county is required to pay for it. Which brings me back to the problem that it will not be paid for unless I give up custody. Obviously, I'm not going to give up custody of my child. It makes me ill that loving parents should be asked such a thing. I feel like this is archaic; are we returning to the dark ages where children who are different are locked away?

The Proper School Setting

Finding the proper school setting is going to be one of your most difficult tasks as a parent. You want your child to thrive and to learn as much as they are capable. The problems arise when you disagree with your child's school on what is a proper school setting. This is the moment when the legal battles begin. Because, unfortunately, if you disagree with your child's school, your only recourse is a legal battle (unless you are dedicated enough to try homeschooling).

Research is a key element to finding the right environment for your child. You will want to live in a county that has a good educational system and the resources available to provide the proper setting for your child.

You will also want to visit your child's future classroom and talk to the teachers there. During your visit you should look for the following:

• A structured environment geared to the special needs of children with autism.

• Rooms with low lighting or non-fluorescent lighting.

• An environment that is flexible to the changing moods and needs of each student.

• Each student is recognized as a unique individual with different strengths and needs.

• A teacher who is open to your input and is willing to try new (even unusual) techniques.

• A small teacher-to-student ratio.

• A class with teacher assistants.

• Teacher must be teaching your child to read, write and do math to the best of your child's abilities. You don't want your child sitting and vegetating all day.

• A class schedule that includes art, music and socialization activities.

• A trampoline, exercise ball, punching bag or other exercise equipment which can be used to relieve stress.

• A couch or mats for relaxation.

• A tent or quiet, low-lit corner where children can go to escape environmental stimuli.

• Opportunities for your child to spend time with non-disabled children.

• A predictable study program.

• A direct, steering educational environment.

• Tasks which are simple, decisive and uniform.

• A behavior strategy that can be agreed upon by both the school and the parent.

The IEP Process

Once your child is found eligible for special education services, an Individualized Education Program (IEP) is written. The IEP contains the services that your child will receive from the school based on your child's current level of functioning. The IEP must contain the following: services your child will receive, where your child will receive these services (known as placement), when the services will begin, how long the services will last, how and when your child's progress will be measured. You have the right to be at the IEP meeting, to bring a legal representative to the meeting, and to have input in the decisions that are made.

Do not sign the IEP unless you are happy with it. If you disagree with the IEP in any way, you have the right to request changes. If the changes are denied you have the right to resolution but you must follow the appropriate procedure:

• Talk with your child's school officials including teachers, evaluators and the principal. Keep accurate and detailed records of your discussions. Your records should include the date and time, who you talked to, and what was discussed. Do not hesitate to bring a recorder to tape meetings—that way there is no question on what is said by whom.
• Request in writing the changes you want made to your child's IEP. Put this in the form of a letter to the principal. Make sure that your letter includes the date, who the letter is addressed to, and your name and address. Send your letter registered so that you have a signature as proof that the letter was received and when it arrived.
• If the principal denies your request you can then move on to a mediation conference to be conducted by an unbiased third party.
• If you are still not satisfied, you have the right to a due process hearing to be conducted in a trial-like setting.
• The next step would be to file a signed, written complaint with you state's department of education.
• If you still do not have the desired result, you may wish to consider legal action against your child's school.

Homeschooling

Homeschooling is a valid option open to you. Check with your county about their individual homeschool laws. There will be forms that you need to fill out and many counties will only accept certain schools that have been pre-approved by the county board of education.

The homeschool you choose will need documentation from your child's doctor showing that he/she is autistic. You will want a homeschool that has advisors and teachers that will guide you in teaching your child.

Homeschooling has many advantages: you avoid the hassles of the IEP process, your child can work at his/her own pace, homeschooled children tend to have higher scores on SOL's and college placement tests. Another advantage of homeschooling is that, through the homeschool, your child may be able to obtain a diploma that is not a special education diploma. I will probably homeschool Jordan during her high school years just for this reason.

Your and Your Child's Rights

Thanks to the Americans With Disabilities Act, your child is guaranteed an education. Public schools are required by law to provide your child with an education that is appropriate and in the least restrictive environment. Your child is also guaranteed the various therapies they need (such as speech, occupation therapy, etc).

Problems arise when parents, doctors, and school officials do not agree on what is an appropriate education. Even though Jordan is now in a special education class, her lawyer is still involved because problems still arise from time to time. Trust me when I say that it is worth the extra money to get a reliable lawyer to have on your side. The school system has lawyers in their employment and they won't think twice to use them.

You must agree to allow the school system to conduct a study on your child. This is called a "child study" and it includes a psychological evaluation, a medical exam, a social history, an educational evaluation, and speech and occupational evaluations. The outcome of their child study rules over all others. It doesn't matter how many private doctors you have on your side—all saying that your child's autism requires certain special accommodations. You child will not receive those accommodations if the outcome of the child study is not in sync with your doctor's evaluations. Now, are you starting to understand why it doesn't hurt to have a lawyer on your side?

Having a legal team on your side can be valuable for a number of reasons. There have been some major court decisions made to the benefit of disabled children and their parents. One such case is that of Karl and Linda Peterson on behalf of their autistic son. The courts found that the school system did not provide an appropriate education for their son.

The Individuals with Disabilities Education Improvement Act-Part B, and the Federal Regulations Governing Special Education

The federal government has set up rules and regulations meant to govern special education while guarding the rights of both the parent and child. While this document is much too long to reprint entirely in this book, it contains important information that needs to be discussed.

"Individuals with Disabilities Education Improvement Act of 2004" (IDEA) is a federal law which governs the education of students with disabilities. IDEA 2004 requires that families be informed of their special education rights, including how families and schools can resolve issues."

Students with disabilities (including autism) are guaranteed a Free Appropriate Public Education (FAPE). The child must be taught in the least restrictive environment (LRE). This means that an autistic child may spend his/her full day in an autism class, or they spend part of the day in a class with non-disabled children. The goal of LRE is to have the child spend as little time as possible in a restrictive environment.

Your child's school must come up with a plan on how your child will be educated. This plan is called the Individualized Education

Program (IEP). You, as the parent, have a right to input your concerns and ideas into the IEP. Your child's school must have consent from you before they can put the IEP in place. The school must also provide you with progress reports. An IEP must include: your child's present level of academic functioning, the aids and special services your child will receive, annual goals, an explanation of the amount of time your child will be in special education classes, accommodations necessary for learning and testing, and a plan for how your child will participate in your state's SOL's or other accountability testing.

You, as the parent, have a right to an interpreter if English is not your first language, or if you are deaf.

"You have the right to be given written information about the school division's actions which involve your child's education needs. The information will assist you in providing informed consent for education decisions."

This statement means that your child's school is required by law to notify you in writing of any changes it plans to make in your child's status as a disabled student, or changes in your child's IEP.

The school must also give you written notice if it refuses to make changes in your child's status as a disabled student, or make changes in your child's IEP. Parents are becoming creative with this section of the law by insisting that their child's school put in writing why it refuses to take into consideration any suggestions the parent may have about improving their child's education plan.

The written notice must include the following:

• Description of the action that your child's school proposes or refuses to take.
• An explanation as to why the action is being proposed or refused.
• Describe each evaluation, report, or assessment the school used in order to reach their decision.
• Include a statement that you have protection under the procedural safeguards provisions in the IDEA
• Tell you how you can obtain a copy of the procedural safeguards.

• Include resources that will help you understand IDEA.
• List all the choices the IEP team considered and why they were rejected.

"You have the right to have information in a language you understand."

This means that an interpreter must be available to you if you do not speak English. If you are deaf, you have the right to a sign language interpreter and communication written in Braille.

"You have certain consent rights. For example, the school must get your consent to evaluate your child for special education, and to start, change, or stop providing special education and related services."

Your child's school must ask your permission before it can:

• Do an evaluation on your child.
• Put your child in a special education class.
• Reevaluate your child.

The school may not deny your child the opportunity to benefit from other services and/or future services because you have denied your consent in the past.

Your child's school does not have to ask for your consent before doing the following:

• Review existing information to reevaluate or evaluate your child.
• Give your child a test or evaluation that is given to all children regardless.

The school can attempt to gain your consent or otherwise seek to do their evaluations or placements without your consent through mediation and "due process."

The school can do their evaluations and/or placement without your consent if they can prove that they have attempted to make contact with the parent and that the parent has ignored their requests. The school is liable to show that they have tried to make contact with you through documentation which includes: detailed records of phone calls, copies of correspondence, and detailed records of visits to the parent's home or place of employment.

"If you disagree with an evaluation completed by the school division, you have the right to have your child evaluated by someone not connected to your child's school division, at the school division's expense."

If the school does an evaluation of your child and you are not happy with the outcome, you have the right to request an independent evaluation at the expense of the school. The big "but" here is that you must follow the criteria outlined by the school. Also, the school will provide you with information about where you can have the evaluation done. This means that you probably will not be allowed to choose your own provider. You have the right to an independent evaluation at public expense. However, to get this you must prove that the school evaluation did not meet its own criteria, or that it was inappropriate for your child.

If, like me, you went out and paid for an independent evaluation on your child, the school must consider this evaluation only if it meets school criteria for an independent evaluation. The criteria for an independent evaluation can vary by state.

"You have the right to be told by the state about how information about your child will be used and kept confidential by the state and the local school division."

"You have the right to review your child's records."

You have a right to review you child's school records. Your child's school has 45 calendar days to grant you this request. You have a right to review your child's records before an IEP meeting. Your legal representative also has the right to review your child's records. The school must also provide you copies of your child's records if you live out of state, are incapacitated, or otherwise unable to visit the school to see the records.

"If your child's education record is seen by someone other than you, or an employee of the school division, the school that maintains your child's record must keep a record of who saw your child's record, and when and why they reviewed it."

Each school must keep a record of parties obtaining access to your child's records including the name of the party given access, the date they looked at the file, and the reason they looked at it.

"You have the right to ask that your child's education record be changed. If you think the record is not correct or that it violates your child's privacy."

You can request that information in your child's file be changed if you think it is incorrect, misleading, or violates your right to privacy. The school must respond to your quest within a "reasonable" amount of time. There is no wording as to the definition of "reasonable." Therefore, the amount of time your school can take is determined by your local board of education.

"You have the right to a hearing if your request to have your child's education record changed is denied."

Upon your request, the school division must provide you the opportunity for a hearing to challenge the information in your child's school records if you feel that the information is incorrect, misleading, or violates your right to privacy.

"You have the right to have your child's education record changed as a result of a hearing or to include a statement in the education record noting that you disagree with information in the record."

If as a result of a hearing, your child's records are determined to be incorrect, misleading, or violating your right to privacy, the school must change the school's records.

If, as a result of the hearing, it is decided that your child's records are not incorrect, misleading or in violation of your right to privacy, you still have the right to make a statement commenting on the information. Your statement must be included as part of your child's record.

"You have the right to ask for mediation to resolve a disagreement, including those issues which lead to a request for a due process hearing. You and the school division have the right to refuse mediation. Your request for mediation cannot slow down or stop your request for due process."

Your child's school must make mediation available if you wish to resolve a dispute without a due process hearing. Mediation must be agreed to by both parties and the outcome of such is legally binding.

"You have the right to ask for a due process hearing if you and the school cannot agree about your child's education. You have the right to receive information about free or low-cost legal help."

If you are not able to settle your dispute with the school through mediation, then you have the right to take your grievance to a court.

"Your request for due process must include certain information. You have the right to have the request kept confidential. You have the right to have a response to your request."

The request for due process must include your child's name and address, the name of the school, facts relating to the problem, and a proposed resolution. The school division has ten calendar days to respond to your request. The school division's response must include an explanation of why the school division refused to take action, other actions that were considered but refused for you child's IEP, and a description of each evaluation and assessment the school used to reach their decisions.

"Except in specialized circumstances, your child has the right to continue getting the same educational services until the due process is resolved, unless you and the school division make a different agreement."

The school cannot change the services your child is receiving until the due process hearing.

"Before a due process hearing is held, you have the right to meet with school staff to discuss the issues in your due process case, and to try to resolve your concerns. However, you and the school division can agree that you both do not want a resolution meeting, or you can both agree to use mediation."

The school division has 15 days to convene a meeting with all relevant members of the IEP team. Important information to remember here is that at this meeting there must be a representative from the school division with decision-making authority, and there cannot be a school attorney present unless you have an attorney present.

"You have certain rights during due process hearings, including the right to have access, before the hearing, to all of the evidence that the school will use during the hearing, to have a lawyer or persons helping you, to have a record of the hearing at no cost, and to have the hearing open to the public."

You have the right to a lawyer, to present evidence and cross-examine witness, to prohibit the introduction of evidence that has not been disclosed five business days before the hearing, and to obtain a written record of the hearing.

"You have the right to have a decision based on the issues in your due process request, to file a separate due process request if new issues arise, and to have information that specifically identifies your child removed from the hearing decision before the decision is made public."

I want to stress here that you have the right to file another due process hearing if new issues come up.

"You have the right to have the hearing at a time and place that is convenient to you, and to have a final decision in the hearing within a set timeline, and to receive a copy of the decision."

"If either you or the school division disagrees with the hearing decision, a civil action can be filed in state or federal court, but there is a time limit."

You have one year from the day of the decision of the due process hearing to file a civil action in state circuit court, or 90 calendar days to file in federal district court.

"A court may decide that the losing party must pay the other party's legal fees."

My strongest advice to everybody dealing with the school system is to get the advice of an attorney who has expertise in dealing with the public school system.

Section 504 of the Rehabilitation Act of 1973

This federal law prohibits schools from discriminating against children with disabilities and requires that schools accommodate the child's needs. It is much easier for the parent to get accommodations under 504 than it is to get services under IDEA. Unlike IDEA, Section 504 does not require a child study and it covers a greater number of children than does IDEA. For example: Let's say that your child has Asperger's but your child's school does not think your child needs to be in a special education class. Under Section 504 your child can receive accommodations such as: longer time to finish tasks, taking tests in a separate room where it is quiet, etc. Section 504 does not cover services such as speech therapy, etc.

Relinquishment of Custody as a Requirement to Obtain Out-of-Home Services

Many parents have had to deal with the unthinkable—giving away their child in order to obtain the medical services that their child needs. This sounds barbaric but it is a common practice in the following states:

Colorado, Indiana, Iowa, Nebraska, Tennessee, West Virginia, Arizona, California, Florida, Illinois, Kentucky, Louisiana, Maryland, Michigan, Missouri, New York, Ohio, Texas, Utah, Connecticut, Kansas, Maine, Minnesota, North Dakota, Oregon, Virginia, Pennsylvania, and Vermont. Researchers have encountered difficulty when attempting to collect data but 25 percent of parents surveyed said that they had been advised to give up custody in order to get services for their child. It is estimated that this problem could potentially affect hundreds of thousands of parents and children.

The spring 2001 edition of the *Journal of Emotional and Behavior Disorder* stated that the loss of parental rights is a fundamental issue and noted the following:

• Differential implementation of custody policies among single-parent families, minorities, and the poor.
• Harmful effects on the parent's self-concept.
• Harmful effects on society's concept of families.
• Negative influences on parent's relationships with social services agencies.
• Erosion of the parent/child relationship.
• Limits a parent's involvement in key decision making regarding their child's health and education.
• Undermines family integrity.
• Keeps the child from sharing in family culture, holidays, religious and family traditions.
• Puts a monetary strain on family welfare agencies.
• Penalizes families for the state's failure to develop adequate services and supports.

The reason for this practice comes down to that nasty little word with a big meaning, "money." Insurance companies will not pay for exorbitant, long-term, or out-of-home care. Most families can not afford to pay the high cost of treatment. Relinquishing custody is a way for welfare services to tap into funds available for orphans, foster care, and special education.

Become Active in Politics

As the parent of a special-needs child you have an even greater responsibility to take an interest in the political scene of your community, county, state, and even on the federal level. You need to know what bills and pieces of legislation could have an impact on your child's life as well as your own. You also need to know how your representatives are voting on these bills. If you are a registered voter, then someone in your representative's office is required to talk to you. You may get an assistant and not your actual senator or House member, but this is okay. Assistants are trained and work closely with your representative. They will give your representative your concerns. In fact, don't just call—make an appointment to come in and visit their office. I have worked for a few lobbying groups, therefore, I feel I am qualified to give a few pointers on how to make your meeting a success.

- Do your research beforehand. Thanks to the Freedom of Information Act, it is public knowledge which bills are coming to the floor (meaning they will be voted on). Your state should have a public website where you can access upcoming bills. If you have trouble finding it, don't hesitate to call your local representative and ask.
- Don't be nervous at the meeting. As a registered voter you hold a certain type of power over your representative. Don't hesitate to say that you will not be voting for this person in the next election if you are not happy with them.
- Dress appropriately in business attire. Dark blues are favorable. Don't wear flashy jewelry or outrageous makeup.
- Speak calmly and clearly.
- Know beforehand what you plan to say and how you are going to say it.
- Make eye contact.
- Be serious—no gigging, loud talking, or laughing (unless your representative makes a joke meant as an ice breaker).
- A firm handshake earns respect.

Chapter 9

We were at an amusement park and we got on a whole bunch of rides and we were trying to find our way out. And, there were a whole bunch of people behind us and even I kept on running away. And we found a whole bunch of people and I finally got lost. Even then I looked everywhere and I looked through all the people. Even then I finally went to the person who worked there and they wouldn't listen to me. And they finally got onto the edge of nerves and they finally understand you. Even then I told them that I got lost. Even they were trying to figure out my mom's name. Even then I said Brenda but they couldn't understand. Even then they said what kind of shirt. Even then I said black stripes. Even then I told them a black car. Even then while my mom was talking to the policeman. He had a microphone. My mom said I bet that is her. Even then my mom got there. Even then we were happy.

Teach kids to go up to somebody who works there and tell them that you are lost. Tell them your name. Even tell them their mommy's shirt. And tell them what kind of shirt or the car. Tell kids not to talk to strangers. And teach them about fireman and policeman and ambulance. And go to a policeman, fireman, or ambulance. Don't be afraid of them. They can help you, right?

—Jordan (recounting her experience of getting lost)

Jordan was having a very bad day. One of her worst: she was being violent and cursing at everyone and everything. It was all I could do to keep her contained. Jordan had consumed my morning and I hadn't had time to deal with anything else. Around noon, a school official called and asked why Jordan was not in school. When I said that she was being violent, the person on the other end of the line asked, "So, does this mean she won't be in school?" I snapped my reply, "Not unless you want to be beaten up." I had surpassed my breaking point.

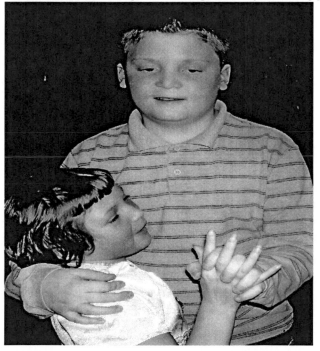

Jordan and her brother Joseph dance together at a family function. The effects of autism and MCDD are felt by the whole family.

Coping Techniques for Parents and Caregivers

Having a disabled child is a 24-hour, 7-days-a-week task. It is tiresome, stressful, sometimes even painful. However, it can also be joyous, wonderful, and delightful. I would not trade one moment of my time with Jordan. However, there are times that I need to walk away and take a break. It is a thin line we walk when caring for a disabled child. It is important that we take care of ourselves as well as we take care of our child.

First and foremost is the need to have a tough skin. Believe me, you will make a few enemies. I am not saying that you should walk around with a chip on your shoulder. Of course, you should be polite and try your hardest to have a good rapport with you child's school and doctors. Unfortunately, the odds are that you will butt heads with someone sooner or later. In researching this book, the one complaint I heard over and over again from people is that it is extremely hard to get their child a good education. If you are the type that tends to steer away from causing any type of opposition, chances are that you are not going to be very successful in your dealings with the public school system.

Other people will be judgmental of you everywhere you go. I often get angry looks from others when Jordan and I are in public. People just assume that she is not disabled. I once had someone in a store come up to me and tell me that Jordan needed a "good old-fashioned spanking." I always tell people that she is autistic. Unfortunately, most people haven't a real clue as to what autism is.

In dealing with the public I find the best thing is to have a sense of humor. I have tried to inform my neighbors of Jordan's disability. One well-meaning neighbor knocked on my door one day to inform me that Jordan had taken off her shoes and was playing in a mud puddle. You should have seen the look on my neighbor's face when I clapped and jumped for joy. Jordan cannot withstand certain textures. She often throws up at the feel of finger paint. Jordan taking off her shoes and playing in the mud was a breakthrough. Unfortunately my neighbor did not understand this.

I think the best piece of advice I have been given came from a dear friend who said to me, "Don't lose yourself for the sake of your children." In other words, don't give up your dreams and your goals in life because you have a disabled child. In fact, I think that now is the perfect time for you to start working towards your goals. I cannot stress this enough. You will be faced with a mountain of challenges and it will be extremely easy to give up on yourself and give your entire being to the care of your child. This sounds like a heroic action; however, the result is going to be that you will be worn out, stressed out, and angry at your child.

Learn to turn negatives into positives. I was forced to quite working full-time in order to meet Jordan's needs. I was not able to find a part-time job that allowed me to work only the hours that Jordan was in school. I began to write at home. Writing is something that I have always said that I would do "someday." Writing fit into my schedule perfectly. I started to write for several websites. And now, less than 18 months later, I am publishing my first book. So, the moral of the story is, stop putting off your goals until "someday." If you do, chances are that "someday" will never come.

Make a daily schedule for yourself and stick to it as much as possible. If you schedule 45 minutes daily for housecleaning but don't get the dusting done, oh well, the dusting can be done the next day.

Meditate daily. This is not hard to do. All you really need is a cheap timer and a quiet place. Light some incense and a candle and just relax your mind for a few minutes. It doesn't have to be long—even five or ten minutes will do. You owe it to yourself to spend a few minutes to rest and not think of anything. You will be surprised at how refreshing this can be.

It is okay to cry. It is okay to have bursts of anger. Release it and then continue on with your life.

Find enjoyment in the little moments. The Buddhist religion teaches "mindfulness," or being in the moment. If you find you are having a joyful moment with your child, or see something beautiful such as a rainbow in the sky (or whatever brings you joy), stop for a moment and be thankful for it.

Spend time with your friends. Go out at least once a month, even if it is just for coffee. Promise yourself that you and your friends will not talk about anything negative during this outing.

Knowledge is power, so do your research. Know everything you can about your child's condition and your legal rights. Have a legal advisor that you can turn to.

If possible cut back your hours at work. Under the Family Medical Leave Law, you are entitled to 40 days of leave (to be used for doctors appointments and therapy appointments). Your place of employment should have the necessary forms for this. It does require that a form be filled out by your child's doctor.

Social Security. The chances are good that your child qualifies for social security benefits. You can use this money so that you can cut back your hours at work. Or use the money to pay for extras that insurance will not cover; such as ballet, equine therapy, etc.

Take time out for yourself. You should not feel guilty for needing a break. Taking a break means that you will come back refreshed and with more energy to give to your child. This is also important for married couples or a caregiver who has a partner. You will need that special time alone to keep your relationship on track. There are respite services available if you are not able to find a family member who is willing to watch your child during your time away from home.

Don't feel guilty. You did nothing to cause your child's autism. Don't be angry at your child. Just as you did not do anything to cause their autism, nor did they do anything to cause it.

Chapter 10

Jordan is my greatest joy. We have spent many magical moments together playing in the surf at the beach, riding roller coasters, and watching her play video games with her brother. One of my greatest concerns evolves around what her future holds. Will she ever marry her prince? Will she slay the bad dragons and save the good ones?

More realistically, I worry about if she will be able to work, hold down a job, and live on her own. What will happen to her when I can no longer watch over her? Will her older brother see her as a burden or will he come to see her as the beautiful person that I know she can be? Will she ever find someone who loves her as much as her family members?

My concerns are valid. And they are problems that will be faced by every parent with an autistic child.

Thanks to the recent breakthrough in gene research, new understanding of autism is on the horizon. This new understanding will eventually lead to new treatments and, hopefully, a cure, but this requires research. This is why we, as citizens, must contact our representatives and demand that more money be given towards this end. The National Institute of Health (NIH) is currently conducting an amazing amount of research on autism. Research which children may participate in for free, including free medications and access to some of the top doctors in the autism field. For this important research to continue, both Congress and the president need to allocate more funding. It is unfortunate that any breakthroughs from stem cell research will not come from this country. It is unfortunate that the Dutch are the only ones doing research on children with multiple complex developmental disorder. The more people we have working on the problem, the more likely it is that we will see a breakthrough. You, as a parent, are not powerless in your influence over your child's future. I cannot stress enough how important it is that you become an active citizen.

Prepare your autistic child for the future just as you do your non-autistic children. Make sure that they receive the best education possible. Teach your child basic life skills such as cooking, cleaning, and how to handle money. Encourage them, encourage them, and then encourage them some more. And don't forget to praise them. Even if they fail at the task, praise them for the attempt. Do everything you can to boost their self-confidence. Enroll them into a variety of sporting activities and artistic activities. It does not take a large amount of money to do this. Most counties will waive park and recreation fees for low-income residents. Many dance and art academies have scholarships. (However, most do not advertise this so you will need to ask). The Special Olympics provides sporting opportunities for free.

The future is full of the unknown. And the way can be murky. But we, like Jordan, must learn to face our fears and find courage. I pray that your child will learn to "walk the forest" and "save the dragons"; just like Jordan.

Lightning Source UK Ltd.
Milton Keynes UK
UKOW02f1115010316

269382UK00001B/40/P